Motherwell Maternity Fitness Plan

Motherwell Maternity Fitness Plan

Bonnie Berk, RN

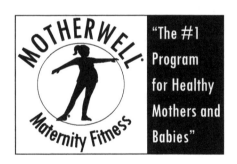

"The #1 Program for Healthy Mothers and Babies"

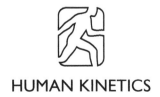

HUMAN KINETICS

Library of Congress Cataloging-in-Publication Information

Berk, Bonnie.
  Motherwell maternity fitness plan / Bonnie Berk.
     p. cm.
  Includes bibliographical references and index.
  ISBN 0-7360-5293-3 (soft cover)
  1. Physical fitness for pregnant women. 2. Exercise for pregnant women. 3. Pregnant women--
Health and hygiene. 4. Mothers--Health and hygiene. I. Title.
  RG558.7.B474 2004
  618.2'44--dc22

                                                                                                2004010390

ISBN-10: 0-7360-5293-3
ISBN-13: 978-0-7360-5293-1

The Web addresses cited in this text were current as of August 2004, unless otherwise noted.

Acquisitions Editor: Martin Barnard; **Developmental Editor:** Cynthia McEntire; **Assistant Editors:** Scott Hawkins, Kim Thoren; **Copyeditor:** Joanna Hatzopoulos Portman; **Proofreader:** Sara Wiseman; **Indexer:** Susan D. Hernandez; **Permission Manager:** Toni Harte; **Graphic Designer:** Robert Reuther; **Graphic Artist:** Francine Hamerski; **Cover Designer:** Keith Blomberg; **Photographer (cover):** Comstock Images; **Art Manager:** Kareema McLendon; **Illustrator**: Argosy; **Printer:** Total Printing Systems

Human Kinetics books are available at special discounts for bulk purchase. Special editions or book excerpts can also be created to specification. For details, contact the Special Sales Manager at Human Kinetics.

Printed in the United States of America   10 9 8 7 6 5 4

The paper in this book is certified under a sustainable forestry program.

Human Kinetics
Website: www.HumanKinetics.com

United States: Human Kinetics
P.O. Box 5076
Champaign, IL 61825-5076
800-747-4457
e-mail: humank@hkusa.com

Canada: Human Kinetics
475 Devonshire Road, Unit 100
Windsor, ON N8Y 2L5
800-465-7301 (in Canada only)
e-mail: info@hkcanada.com

Europe: Human Kinetics
107 Bradford Road
Stanningley
Leeds LS28 6AT, United Kingdom
+44 (0)113 255 5665
e-mail: hk@hkeurope.com

Australia: Human Kinetics
57A Price Avenue
Lower Mitcham, South Australia 5062
08 8372 0999
e-mail: info@hkaustralia.com

New Zealand: Human Kinetics
P.O. Box 80
Torrens Park, South Australia 5062
0800 222 062
e-mail: info@hknewzealand.com

This book is dedicated to all the women who have allowed me to touch their lives, to all of my teachers for helping me find my path, and to my wonderful family for supporting me through this and all of my endeavors.

contents

preface ix

acknowledgments xiii

introduction xv

Chapter 1 **Shaping Up Before Pregnancy** 1
Assessing Health Before Conception ▪ Exercising to Manage Stress ▪
Conditioning the Core ▪ Improving Flexibility ▪ Cooling Down

Chapter 2 **Caring for Your Body During All Nine Months** 21
Getting Relief From Common Discomforts ▪ Posturing for a Healthy
Pregnancy ▪ Protecting Your Back ▪ Going Easy on Your Feet ▪
Taking Care of Your Teeth ▪ Caring for Your Breasts ▪ Caring for Your
Skin ▪ Taking Time for You

Chapter 3 **Breathing Routines for Two** 45
Understanding Belly Breathing ▪ Breathing Exercises ▪ Take a Breath!

Chapter 4 **Eating for Fitness and Baby's Health** 53
Gaining an Appropriate Amount of Weight ▪ Nutritional Considerations
for Vegetarians ▪ Foods to Avoid During Pregnancy

Chapter 5 **Stretching and Strengthening
Your Pregnant Body** 65
Maternal Responses to Exercise ▪ Physiological Considerations ▪
Symptoms of Overtraining ▪ Exercise Safety ▪ Popular Recreational
Exercises and Sports ▪ The Pregnant Athlete ▪ Everyday Stretches ▪
Strengthening Muscles to Support Your Baby ▪ Workout Schedule

Chapter 6 **Meditating for Relaxation and Focus** 103
Getting Started ▪ Meditation Exercises ▪ Preparing for Labor Meditation

Chapter 7   **Adjusting Actively to the First Trimester** 111
Tips for the First Trimester ▪ Exercising on a Fitness Ball

Chapter 8   **Staying Motivated Through
the Second Trimester** 123
Stay Off Your Back ▪ Reclaiming Your Energy ▪ Counting Fetal
Movements ▪ Understanding Premature Labor ▪ Making Love During
Pregnancy

Chapter 9   **Staying Positive in the Third Trimester** 131
Thinking Positively ▪ Exercising With a Chair ▪ Sciatica in Pregnancy ▪
Pros and Cons of Episiotomy ▪ Perineal Massage ▪ Making a Birth Plan

Chapter 10   **Training for Labor and Delivery** 153
Discomfort During Labor ▪ Exercises to Cope With Labor ▪ Massage ▪
Music ▪ Ready, Get Set, It's Labor Time!

Chapter 11   **Adjusting During the Early Weeks
After Delivery** 171
Staying Well Nourished ▪ Proper Body Mechanics for the New Mom ▪
Exercising After Delivery ▪ Getting to Know Your Newborn ▪
Infant Massage

Chapter 12   **Fitness for the New Mom** 183
Sexual Health After Delivery ▪ Exercising After the First Month
Postpartum ▪ Exercising With Baby ▪ Lifetime Fitness for the Whole
Family

bibliography 203
index 205
about the author 213

preface

Giving birth is one of the greatest miracles on earth. It can also be one of the most difficult challenges in a woman's life if she is not physically or mentally prepared. Many unknowns surround pregnancy and childbirth, and women who eat sensibly, exercise regularly, and take the time to learn important coping strategies are more likely to have positive pregnancy and postpartum experiences.

In 1980, I was a labor and delivery room nurse, teaching childbirth classes in one of the largest teaching hospitals in Philadelphia. A large majority of pregnant women in my classes complained of backaches, headaches, anxiety, depression, and various other common discomforts of pregnancy. Many felt guilty about gaining too much weight and felt out of shape.

At that time, I had an idea that if these women exercised and spent time with other pregnant women focusing on the positive aspects of pregnancy, they would feel better, look better, and have a better attitude toward their pregnancies and their expanding waistlines. I developed a fitness class that combined both exercise and health education with the goal of preparing women's minds and bodies for pregnancy, delivery, and the postpartum period. Hence, Motherwell was born!

Twenty-five years ago, very little was known about exercise during pregnancy. In fact, most obstetricians recommended that pregnant women avoid exercise, unless they were exercising prior to pregnancy. Current research, however, shows that there are more risks from not exercising during pregnancy than exercising on a regular basis. The benefits of exercise for both mom and baby are discussed in chapter 5.

Obesity is an epidemic in our society, resulting in a high incidence of heart disease, high blood pressure, and diabetes. In pregnancy, obesity is a major predictor of poor pregnancy outcome. To reduce the chance of having a high-risk pregnancy, women are urged to practice healthy lifestyles even before pregnancy. The first chapter of this book discusses the importance of *Shaping Up Before Pregnancy* and offers many suggestions for enhancing your health to better support fetal growth and development. Fetal development is crucial in the early months of gestation. Women exposed to high temperatures early in pregnancy can have babies with birth defects. The same is true for women with vitamin and nutritional deficiencies. Unfortunately, many women do not even know they are pregnant until the end of the first trimester. That is why women need to consciously prepare for pregnancy and adopt healthy lifestyles while they are trying to conceive.

Initially, when I began the Motherwell program, not many women were exercising on a regular basis and I had to convince both health care providers and their patients alike of the benefits of exercise during pregnancy. Now, the pendulum has swayed in the other direction! Many young women are not only exercising, but performing more strenuous exercise as well as dieting obsessively. The old adage of "continuing what you did before pregnancy" just isn't appropriate for these women when they become pregnant. In fact, many women who exercise strenuously and diet excessively have a difficult time becoming pregnant at all. The same is true for women who have stressful lifestyles and poor coping skills. That is why it is recommended that these women also modify their lifestyles prior to pregnancy, being sure to eat nutritiously, exercise moderately, and learn ways to cope with stress.

The Motherwell Fitness Program is intended for the average healthy woman with no chronic disease or acute illness. Be sure to consult your health care provider prior to starting this or any exercise program. For health and fitness professionals, this book provides a great resource for working with patients and clients. For questions on developing group fitness classes, or specific situations, please email me at bonnie@bonnieberk.com.

This book offers easy-to-follow strategies for exercise, diet, and modifying your lifestyle in order to have a healthy pregnancy and a satisfying postpartum experience. There are also suggestions for preventing and/or alleviating the common discomforts of pregnancy, from nausea and fatigue in the early days of pregnancy, to pelvic pressure and low back discomfort in the latter months of pregnancy.

Sexual health plays an important role in the overall well-being of women and their partners. In both men and women, having a healthy sex life can contribute to a strong immune system as well as the health of the reproductive organs. It is not uncommon for couples to have relationship problems due to sexual issues during pregnancy and the postpartum phase. Studies show that many marriages break up within a year after the birth of a baby. This book offers important strategies for developing positive communication with your partner as well as suggestions on how to keep sexually active throughout your pregnancy and after delivery.

Several chapters focus on preparing the mind and body for the labor and delivery experience. Chapter 10 also provides the expectant mom with useful tools for getting through childbirth in the most positive ways possible and describes the best exercises for comfort during labor and delivery.

Usually exercise is the last thing on most women's minds after delivery. However, exercise, proper nutrition, and adequate rest are essential in reducing the risk of postpartum depression. New moms are encouraged to gradually ease back into exercise while adjusting to the role of new parent. For women who want to get rid of those excess pounds after delivery, there is a sensible eating plan for both breast- and bottle-feeding moms.

Parents find that their children imitate them in more ways than they care to envision sometimes. Children will do as you do more often than they will do as you say. By practicing a healthful lifestyle while you are pregnant, and continuing after delivery, you set a healthful example for your children. The benefits are more far reaching than you can ever imagine!

Get started today! If you are pregnant or thinking about getting pregnant, this book will provide you with everything you need to stay fit and healthy before, during and after pregnancy. Best wishes for a happy and healthy pregnancy!

acknowledgments

Many thanks go to the wonderful people who believed in me over the years and shared in my vision. I especially want to thank Gerri George for helping me in the early days.

I also want to thank Dr. Al Paolone and Dr. Mona Shangold for sharing their time and expertise. Thanks to Dr. Karen Glanz, who took the time and effort to oversee the design of a research project proving the benefits of the Motherwell program.

At a time when many obstetricians were cautious about recommending exercise to pregnant women, Dr. Ronald Librizzi supported my endeavors and continually gave me words of encouragement.

As with any career, I have had my share of ups and downs. Thanks to my lawyer, Carol Lindsay, who gave me the courage to stick it out when the going got rough.

When I wanted to make the *Motherwell Yoga Video for Expectant Moms*, Ernie Lavasseur provided me with the financial help and guidance I needed to complete the project. And thanks to Herb Rosenbaum for designing a spectacular Web site and guiding me through the computer maze.

I am fortunate to have met some amazing women who supported my work and helped sustain me over the years. Thanks to Karen Harkins, Camille Baughman, Jacqueline Powell, Rita Schlansky, Deborah Snelson, Eileen Swidler, Judy Perlman, and Tracy Wood. Thanks to Petra Wirth for being my mentor and friend. My sincere appreciation also goes to my friend and assistant, Melissa Brehm.

In loving memory, I want to thank Larry Patullo, a friend and my first video producer, and Sylvia Olkin, who was my inspiration for developing the Motherwell Yoga Program.

Special thanks to my husband, Ted, and children, Liz, Emily, and Ben, for giving me inspiration, joy, and frequent back rubs after I sat at the computer for long hours. Thanks to my cat, Buddy, and my dog, Sage, for their companionship while I worked in my home office. And thanks to my parents, Melvin and Corinne Fischman, for showing me how to enjoy life!

introduction

When people hear the word *fitness*, it usually conjures up visions of young, buff bodies pumping iron in a gym. But the face of fitness has changed for the better over the years. In the early 1980s, fitness was about getting your body to look a certain way, regardless of how you felt. Today, the focus of fitness is to prepare your body for functional activities, to avoid injury, and to gain an overall sense of well-being.

Today, when professionals talk about fitness, they are not only referring to physical fitness, but to mental and emotional fitness as well. The term *mind–body fitness* refers to this holistic philosophy. We are more than just a physical shell to be molded and chiseled into shape. Everything affects our bodies, even our thoughts!

Mind affects body and body affects mind. The science of psychoneuroimmunology is the medical field of investigation that studies the relationship of the mind to the body and its effect on health and disease. In ancient times, Hippocrates, the father of Western medicine, taught his students to look at psychosocial factors surrounding individuals to help understand certain diseases. Yet, it has been fairly recent that the scientific community seriously considered the notion of mind–body unity and its effect on health and well-being.

Over the last decade, researchers have shown a relationship between stress and a wide variety of diseases. Affective states such as depression have been shown to lower immune function. There is also evidence that the way a person perceives a stressful event impacts on immune function. In fact, perception of an illness has been shown to affect the course of diseases such as cancer and human immunodeficiency virus (HIV) infection.

Researchers have shown that there is a pathway of communication called the hypothalamus-pituitary-adrenal axis (HPA) on which the central nervous system and endocrine system exchange signals. These communications are bidirectional and cause a series of complex cellular changes. Chemical transmitters allow thoughts and emotions to stimulate sensory and motor neurons as well as glandular tissue and immune cells.

Glucocorticoids secreted from the adrenal cortex in times of stress tend to decrease immune function. Other stress hormones, catecholamines, and neuropeptides, which are secreted by the sympathetic nervous system, also suppress immune function as well as affect virtually every system of the body.

The science of psychoneuroimmunology has brought credibility to the notion that thoughts, feelings, and behavior have a direct impact on health. Health care providers are increasingly becoming partners with their patients in preventing and treating diseases. The more known about the mind–body connection, the more choices people have for practicing behaviors that positively impact their health, and in the case of pregnancy, the health of the growing fetus.

However, not every disease or outcome can be avoided by practicing healthful behaviors. Many variables affecting your health and the health of your offspring, such as genetics, environment, and health-protective resources (for example, vaccines), are out of your control. Rather than focus on what you can't control, focus on those factors you can control. Decisions you make every day affect your body.

For example, your food choice has a significant impact on how you feel emotionally as well as on your physical health. Food affects mood. Become aware of how certain foods might affect you. Avoid those foods that make you feel nervous or upset. Avoid foods that make you feel unwell. You wouldn't put cheap gas in a Mercedes. Treat your body as though it were your most valuable possession (it is!). Fill your "gas tank" with the "highest octane" to go the distance.

Whether or not to exercise is a choice that affects all aspects of health. Studies prove that exercise elevates mood, improves circulation, decreases blood pressure, and enhances immune function. In pregnancy, exercise has been shown to decrease the incidence of gestational diabetes and most recently, preeclampsia. Practicing stress management techniques and having positive relationships with those closest to you also have an impact on your health and the health of your unborn baby.

Holistic living is based on the philosophy that everything in life affects health in one way or another. A famous psychologist, Gestalt, once said, "The whole is greater than the sum of its parts." What this means is that when you practice healthful behaviors, the results are farther reaching than your original intent. Maybe you stopped smoking cigarettes to have healthier lungs or to prepare for a healthy pregnancy. Then you found out that without smoking, you have more energy and breath to exercise. And when you exercise, you are more aware of the foods you eat as well as the people in your life. One behavior affects a whole string of behaviors. When you practice healthful behaviors, you also become an inspiration to those around you, including your family.

In the 21st century, achieving fitness means bringing balance into your body and into your life. When your body is not balanced, your health is affected. When your life is out of balance, you can feel it in your body. So, the goal of fitness is to reveal balance in your body on all levels—physical, mental, and emotional.

Spend a few minutes thinking about how you feel, inside and out. Make a list of any symptoms you are experiencing and see whether you can identify any imbalances that feed those symptoms. You will notice that physical imbalance creates mental and emotional imbalance and vice versa.

When imbalances are present in your body prior to pregnancy, chances are that pregnancy will exacerbate those imbalances. If you are struggling in a relationship with your partner, chances are you will become more frustrated as your pregnancy progresses. If you have a bad back from a previous injury, then most likely your backache will worsen during pregnancy.

Taking care of imbalances in your body and in your life before you become pregnant will give you a better chance of having a positive pregnancy and parenting experience. However, if you are already pregnant, it's not too late to start practicing healthful behaviors. So, let's get started.

chapter 1

Shaping Up Before Pregnancy

So, you're thinking about having a baby. That's a good thing. Unfortunately, many women become pregnant without even knowing when and where it happened, and with very little preparation. The health of the mother before she becomes pregnant has a significant impact on the outcome of pregnancy.

Through research, we know that fetal development in the first few months of pregnancy is crucial to the health of the newborn. Alcohol ingested at this time can cause emotional disabilities as well as mental retardation in the child. Cigarette smoking can negatively affect the developing child's cardiovascular health. Lack of certain minerals and vitamins, such as folic acid, may result in birth defects. The good news is that if a woman changes her lifestyle to one that is more conducive to a healthy pregnancy *before* she gets pregnant, the baby has a better chance of avoiding these unnecessary complications.

Although many things during the childbearing years cannot be controlled, many things can be controlled. This chapter focuses on assessing your health status and identifying lifestyle behaviors that you can modify or change to prepare for a healthy pregnancy and positive pregnancy experience.

Assessing Health Before Conception

Seeing your health care provider before becoming pregnant is a good way to start planning for pregnancy. Ask your provider about any regular medications you take and whether you should continue these medications while you are trying to become pregnant. Also, ask about any potential genetic risks related to your background or age at the time you become pregnant. If your health care provider thinks you have a higher-than-normal risk of having a baby with a genetic disorder, you might want to consider genetic counseling as well.

Become aware of your nutritional habits. Be sure to take a multivitamin while you are trying to conceive. Many obstetrical health care providers recommend taking prenatal vitamins during this time to be sure you are getting all that you need to support a healthy pregnancy. In addition to supplements, eat lots of fruits and vegetables and choose breads that are high in fiber and whole grains. Figure 1.1 shows the food pyramid of healthful foods and recommended amounts to include in your diet.

If you smoke cigarettes, consider taking a smoking cessation class before becoming pregnant, because once you become pregnant, it may be more difficult to stop. Alcohol is another substance you might want to avoid while trying to conceive. Talk to your health care provider regarding these and other habits that may negatively affect your pregnancy.

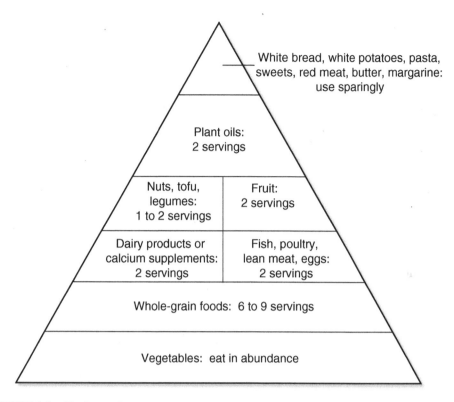

White bread, white potatoes, pasta, sweets, red meat, butter, margarine: use sparingly

Plant oils: 2 servings

Nuts, tofu, legumes: 1 to 2 servings

Fruit: 2 servings

Dairy products or calcium supplements: 2 servings

Fish, poultry, lean meat, eggs: 2 servings

Whole-grain foods: 6 to 9 servings

Vegetables: eat in abundance

FIGURE 1.1 Motherwell prepregnancy food pyramid: recommended daily consumption.

You should also consider getting vaccines before you become pregnant. If you never had the chicken pox, getting the vaccine before becoming pregnant could prevent risks of contracting the disease during your pregnancy. Your health care provider can take a simple blood test to check whether or not you are immune to this as well as other communicable diseases.

Question: What about getting booster shots?

Answer: According to the Centers for Disease Control and Prevention (CDC), all women contemplating pregnancy should receive a tetanus-diphtheria (Td) booster if they have not had one in the last 10 years.

Try to get any Xrays, dental work, or diagnostic tests such as mammography before you get pregnant. Once you become pregnant, many of these tests are not compatible with a healthy pregnancy.

Your partner's health is also important in considering risk factors during pregnancy. He needs to understand the importance of certain lifestyle changes that may affect you and the baby. An example is smoking cigarettes. Studies show that secondhand smoke can actually be more toxic to those around the smoker than to the smoker himself.

Bringing your partner to a pre-conception visit with your health care provider might help dispel any misconceptions about the importance of practicing healthful lifestyle habits as well as give him an opportunity to understand the importance of supporting you through this very special time in both of your lives. It is also easier to make lifestyle changes when partners do it together!

Exercising to Manage Stress

There are various theories regarding the causes of infertility. Stress is one of them. Stress is also believed to contribute to problems throughout pregnancy as well as in labor and delivery. Learning skills to decrease stress before pregnancy can not only help you get pregnant, but make pregnancy and parenting a more pleasant experience. Attend a yoga class and practice relaxation breathing techniques such as those discussed in depth in chapter 6.

Exercise is a proven stress reliever. Taking walks on most days of the week will elevate your mood and prepare your body for the changes that occur in pregnancy. If you are already exercising, then it is recommended that you walk or engage in aerobic exercise 30 to 45 minutes a day at a pace at which you can comfortably talk. However, if you are new to exercise, take it slowly. Start walking 10 to 15 minutes twice a day and build up slowly. Here are 10 tips to help maximize the benefits of walking and get you started:

1. Start in good body alignment and try to maintain correct posture for the duration of the walk. Stand tall with shoulders over hips. Keep your ears aligned with your shoulders and your chin tucked in so the neck is in proper alignment with the spine.

2. Try to keep your abdominal muscles firm by pulling your belly button toward the spine (pull in and up). Breathe into the sides of the torso and into your back.

3. Relax the shoulders and breathe comfortably. The optimal pace is one that allows you to talk but not sing.

4. Stay mindful of what you are thinking about while walking. Try to focus on your breathing and notice how your body feels. Imagine yourself getting healthier, leaner, and stronger.

5. Stretch after walking, especially the muscles of your legs. Stretch the calves, quadriceps, and hamstrings. Lower back stretches are also helpful in preventing back discomfort.

6. Wear comfortable shoes with good arch support. Make sure that your shoes have enough toe room so when you step, you are not jamming your toes into the front of the shoe.

7. While walking, listen to relaxing music or a book on tape to add variety and enjoyment to your exercise.
8. Dress appropriately for the weather. Layer clothing on cooler days, and take off outer layers as your body starts to warm up.
9. Discover new paths. Life is a journey. Try walking in different directions and in varied settings. Find out where hiking trails are in your area. Keep your journey as interesting as possible.
10. Make walking a habit. The most important tip for getting the benefits of walking is to make a long-term commitment. Try to integrate walking opportunities into your day. Some suggestions include parking your car farther away from your destination or taking a walk while visiting with a friend.

Other aerobic activities include swimming, biking, dancing, and running. You may also continue attending fitness classes, but try to exercise at a moderate intensity. High internal body temperature during the early weeks of pregnancy may contribute to birth defects of the spine. It is also a good idea to limit your time in hot tubs and saunas.

In addition to walking or engaging in an aerobic activity, you need to strengthen key muscles and improve flexibility to avoid injury and discomfort once you become pregnant. Plan to stretch every day. If you are involved in a weight training program, you may stick with your regimen, but rather than trying to build strength, work to maintain what you have already accomplished. Reduce the amount of weight you are lifting and increase the number of repetitions.

If you are not currently engaged in any strength or flexibility program, the following exercises will help you gain strength and endurance for one of the most important events in your life. Even if you are already taking an exercise class or doing strength and flexibility exercises, add these to your routine.

Conditioning the Core

The *core* is the central part of the body and consists of all the muscles that support the spine. *Stability* refers to the capacity of the body to maintain or return to a state of equilibrium.

The deep muscles of the spine and the abdominal muscles that support the spine react quickly to changes in movement and usually respond first to keep the spine in alignment. This is what it means to *move from the core.* When the core muscles are working effectively, the recruitment of deep muscle fibers for stabilization occurs automatically.

Unfortunately, repetitive strain and injury as well as weak abdominal muscles cause the body to develop movement patterns to protect the injured muscles and restore equilibrium. So, instead of stimulating the deep muscles to provide stability to the spine, the nervous system compensates for weaknesses by recruiting the superficial muscles. This can lead to muscular tension and further injury, and it can weaken the core.

To change this pattern, an individual needs to increase awareness of body movements and move the spine slowly and consciously. This activates the movement centers of the brain and helps to retrain the deep muscles to become the first responders in establishing core stability.

During pregnancy, the weight of the growing uterus causes the spine to overload every day. The stretching pelvis adds risk of injury to the spine, further weakening core muscles. Building core stability is absolutely essential before, during, and after pregnancy to prevent back injury and improve comfort and function.

Strengthening muscles that support the core before pregnancy is especially important because abdominal muscles stretch in pregnancy and there is no concrete evidence that you can effectively strengthen a stretched muscle.

Belly Breathing

Comfortably sit, stand, or lie on your back. Keep a neutral spine and take a deep breath, expanding the belly. As you exhale, pull the belly button toward the spine. Repeat the exercise12 times, then rest and repeat it 12 more times. Try to practice this exercise throughout the day when you are sitting in traffic or waiting in line at the grocery store.

Rounded Cat Stretch

Get on your knees and hands into a tabletop position. Check your lower back with your hands to make sure it is straight. Take a breath. As you exhale, tighten your abdominal muscles, perform a posterior pelvic tilt, and slowly round up the back, tucking in your chin (figure 1.2).

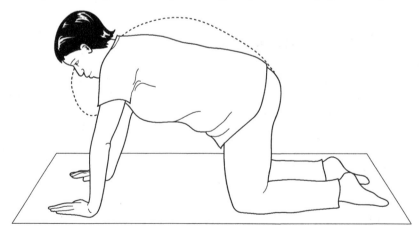

Figure 1.2   Rounded cat stretch: exhale and round the back.

As you inhale, bring the back to a "hollow cat back" by slightly lowering the waist while keeping the abdomen firm. Continue this exercise for 12 breath cycles, then rest with the buttocks on the heels and the arms stretched out above the crown of the head (child's pose; see figure 3.1 on page 48). Repeat the exercise for another 12 breath cycles.

Question: When I exercise on all fours, my wrists bother me. What modifications do you recommend?

Answer: Wrist sensitivity is very common during pregnancy because of the increase in fluid retention. Also some women just seem to have sensitive wrists. To reduce the discomfort in your wrists, make a fist and rest your upper body on the backs of your hands instead of placing your palms flat on the floor. You can also modify the exercise by lowering your body onto your forearms.

Flamingo

Stand in good posture. Take the arms out to the sides at shoulder level and step forward onto the left leg. Bend the right knee behind you and balance (figure 1.3). Keep the abdomen engaged to support the torso and reduce arching of the lumbar spine. Hold this position for 3 to 5 breath cycles. Return to standing position and repeat the exercise on the other side. Repeat one more time on both sides. To make it more challenging, reach the arms overhead with the palms together when you step forward.

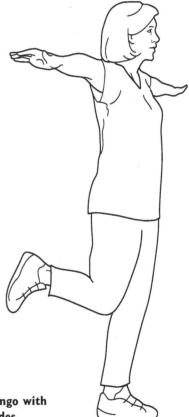

FIGURE 1.3 Flamingo with the arms to the sides.

Balancing Sunbird

Start in a tabletop position with your back flat. Feel with one of your hands to make sure there is no curve in the lower back. Stretch the right leg behind you. Keeping the back straight, raise the heel to the level of the buttocks or below (figure 1.4a). Keep the abdominal muscles engaged to support the lower back and hold the position for 3 to 5 breaths. Bring the right leg in and repeat the exercise with the left leg. Bring left leg in and rest in child's pose (see figure 3.1 on page 48).

Go back into the tabletop position and straighten the right leg behind you, raising the heel to the level of the buttocks or below. Shift your weight onto the right hand and straighten the left arm next to your left ear (figure 1.4b). If this is too difficult, rest your right foot on the floor. Balance in this position while you continue to breathe normally for 3 to 5 breath cycles. Use the muscles of the abdomen to support your back. Bring the leg and arm in and repeat the exercise on the opposite side. Rest in child's pose.

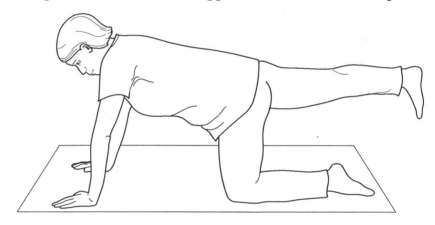

FIGURE 1.4a   Balancing sunbird: raise the right leg.

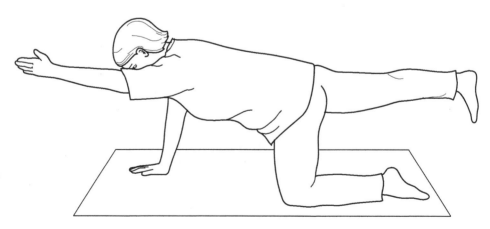

FIGURE 1.4b   Balancing sunbird: raise the right leg and left arm.

Half Crescent Moon

From tabletop position, straighten your left leg behind you and lift the heel to the level of the buttocks or below. Shift your weight onto the right hand and lift the left arm out to the side and up to the ceiling, rotating the body so the left knee and toes are pointing to the left and the left hip is on top of the right (figure 1.5a). Hold this position for 3 to 5 breaths.

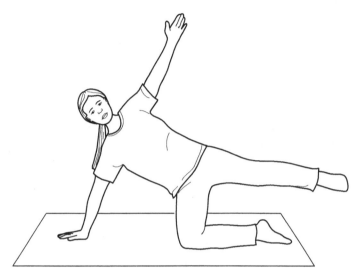

FIGURE 1.5a   Half crescent moon: rotate the body.

Place the left foot back on the floor as you raise the left arm next to the ear and breathe into the left side of the body for 3 to 5 breaths (figure 1.5b). Raise your left arm and left leg again, turn the body toward the floor, and return to tabletop position. Rest in child's pose and repeat the exercise on the right side.

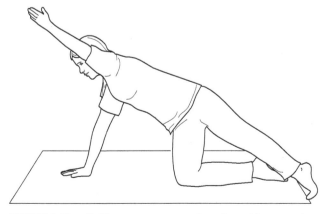

FIGURE 1.5b   Half crescent moon: kneeling side stretch.

Lying Spinal Twists

Lie on your back with knees bent toward the chest and arms out to the sides at shoulder level. Inhale and take the knees over to the side without letting them touch the floor and turn head in opposite direction (figure 1.6). Exhale and bring the knees back to center, moving head back to center. Inhale and bring the knees to the opposite side without the knees touching the floor. Exhale and bring them back to center. Continue moving the knees side to side with the breath for 12 cycles. Rest, then repeat the exercise on each side, allowing the knees to touch the floor to stretch the hips.

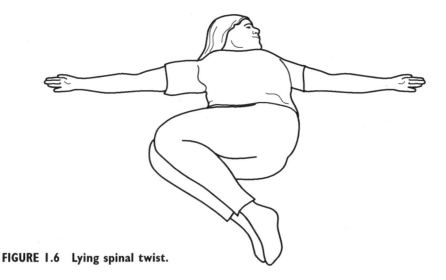

FIGURE 1.6   Lying spinal twist.

Keep the upper body relaxed during the entire exercise. Shoulders should stay on the floor at all times. If you feel any discomfort in the lower back, make the movement smaller. For variation, interlace the fingers and place the hands behind the head. While bringing the knees side to side, keep the elbows on the floor at all times.

Sitting Spinal Twists

Sit comfortably on a chair or on the floor. Keep the back straight with the abdominal muscles engaged. Do not lean back on the chair. Stretch the arms overhead, bringing the palms together and hooking the thumbs. Your arms should be pressing on your ears. If not, tuck the chin in more to bring the head between the arms. Feel a stretch from the hips to the fingertips.

Extend the arms out to the sides at shoulder level as you turn the torso to the right (figure 1.7). Continue to breathe deeply and rhythmically for 3 to 5 breaths. Turn the torso back to center, bringing the arms overhead. Then, rest your hands on your thighs. Stretch the arms overhead again with the palms together. Open the arms out to shoulder level and turn the torso to the left. Hold the position for 3 to 5 breaths and then return to center. Repeat the exercise on each side, resting the arms in between sides. If you experience any shoulder discomfort when stretching with arms up beside ears, then keep arms parallel to each other.

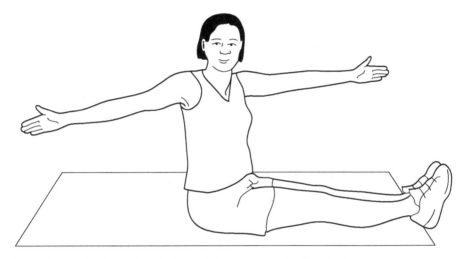

FIGURE 1.7   Sitting spinal twist: rotate the torso to the right.

Kegel Exercises

To build core strength, you also need to strengthen the pelvic floor. Kegel exercises strengthen the pelvic muscles, and stronger pelvic muscles help prevent urine leakage during and after pregnancy as well as restore muscle tone after delivery. Kegels are the most important exercises you will ever do. Many pregnant women who avoid strengthening these muscles tend to experience bowel and bladder incontinence problems later in life.

Take a deep breath and, while exhaling, squeeze the muscles around the vaginal opening and hold. When contracting these muscles, imagine pulling the vaginal opening up toward the inside of the navel. Inhale and release the contraction. Repeat the exercise at least 20 times, twice a day, as if holding something with your vaginal muscles, but feel free to do more. You can never do too many Kegels!

Improving Flexibility

Flexibility refers to joint range of movement as well as the ability of the body to adapt to movement without injury. To become more flexible and maintain flexibility, practice stretching exercises on a daily basis, especially before, during, and after exercise.

Stretching before exercise allows the muscles to warm up in preparation for vigorous activity. As you stretch, more blood flow is brought to the working muscles. Stretching the working muscles after each exercise decreases discomfort and enhances your ability to sustain good form while exercising. After each exercise session, stretching helps prevent muscle soreness and injury and enhances muscle recovery.

As pregnancy progresses, the increased weight of the uterus tends to put stress on the back muscles as well as on the muscles in the hips and groin. The more flexible you are before pregnancy, and the more you maintain your flexibility, the more comfortable you will be throughout pregnancy and the postpartum period. Good flexibility also helps decrease discomfort during labor and delivery.

When practicing exercises to improve flexibility, listen to your body. Stretch muscles slowly and steadily. Avoid bouncing or moving quickly. If you feel any pain or major discomfort as you stretch a muscle, back off and rest. Stretching a tight muscle should feel comfortably uncomfortable. During each stretch, take deep breaths and imagine oxygen traveling to the muscle and helping to release tension. Hold each stretch for 3 to 5 breath cycles and then take note of how you feel.

Leg Extensions

Sit in good posture with the legs extended in front and the hands at the sides. Keep the feet flexed. Lengthen your spine as you inhale and release forward as you exhale, bending from the hip joint, not the waist (figure 1.8). Keep reaching the arms forward and hold the stretch for 3 to 5 breaths. You should feel the stretch behind the knees and in the hamstrings, not the lower back.

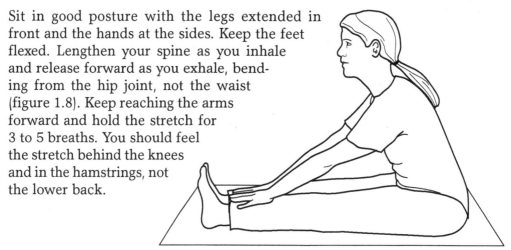

FIGURE 1.8   Leg extension.

Quadriceps Stretch

Lie on your side or stand. Bend one knee and reach back with the hand on the same side to grab the ankle or foot. Gently pull the knee back to stretch the front of the thigh (figure 1.9a). Hold the position for 3 to 5 breaths. Repeat the stretch on the other side. If you feel any pain in the knee-cap, release the stretch and try lying on your side (figure 1.9b). You also can use a strap or piece of cloth to help you reach the ankle.

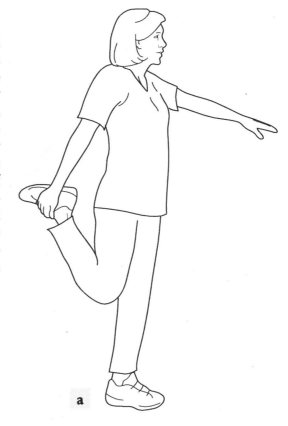

a

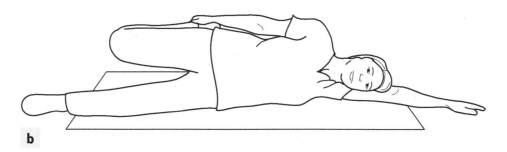

b

FIGURE 1.9   Quadriceps stretch: *(a)* while standing; *(b)* while lying on one side.

Hip Flexor/Monkey Stretch

Kneel on both knees. If this is uncomfortable, roll a towel or blanket under the knees for extra padding. Bring the right foot forward a little farther than the right knee. Interlace your fingers on top of the right knee (figure 1.10). Inhale, lifting up through the torso, and shift your weight forward. Hold the position for 3 to 5 breaths. Repeat the stretch on the other side.

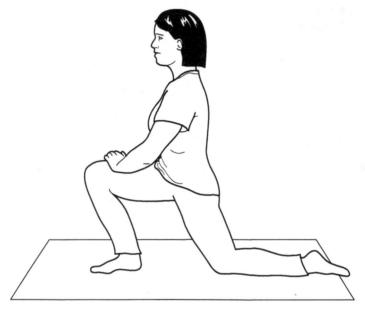

FIGURE 1.10   Hip flexor/monkey stretch.

Squatting

From a tabletop position, separate your feet more than hip-width apart and walk your hands toward the knees while shifting your weight onto the heels of the feet. Either keep your hands on the floor for balance or bring your palms together in front of the heart with the elbows pressing against the inner knees (figure 1.11). Hold the position for 3 to 5 breaths.

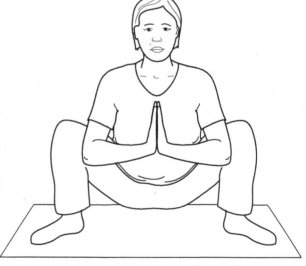

FIGURE 1.11   Squatting.

Shoulder Stretch

Reach behind your back and either hold opposite wrists or interlace the fingers. Bring the palms together and pull the shoulders down and back (figure 1.12). Hold the position for 3 to 5 breaths.

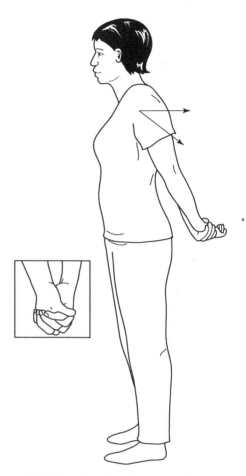

FIGURE 1.12   Shoulder stretch.

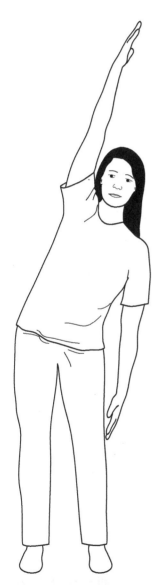

FIGURE 1.13   Standing torso stretch.

Standing Torso Stretch

Stand in good posture, with both arms down at the sides. Inhale and stretch the left arm up to the ceiling. Exhale and lean the torso to the right while sliding the right hand down the outer thigh (figure 1.13). Hold the position for 3 to 5 breaths. Repeat the stretch on the other side.

Garland Pose

From the tabletop position, shift your weight onto the balls of your feet. Extend the arms between the knees (figure 1.14). Hold the stretch for 3 to 5 breaths.

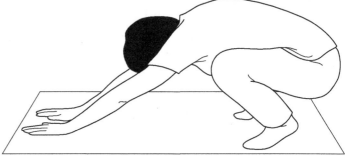

FIGURE 1.14 Garland pose.

Wall-Supported Back Stretch

Lean your hips against a wall with your heels about 6 inches away from the wall. Relax the arms by your sides. As you exhale, bring your chin toward your chest and slowly peel your back off the wall (figure 1.15). Continue to breathe normally. Each time you exhale, try to stretch a little bit further. Do this for 3 to 5 breath cycles. Then as you exhale, tighten your abdomen and slowly bring your upper body back onto the wall, starting at the base of your spine and slowly working up toward the head. Repeat this sequence 3 times.

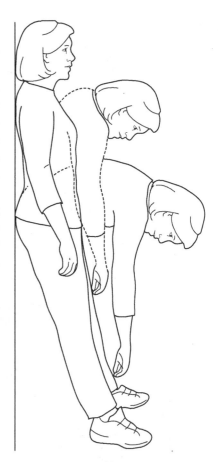

FIGURE 1.15 Wall-supported back stretch.

Standing Forward Bend

Stand in good posture. Exhale and bend the knees slightly. Bring the chin to your chest and slowly roll down toward the floor (figure 1.16). Continue to breathe normally for 3 to 5 breath cycles. With each exhalation, try to get your hands closer to the floor. After 3 to 5 breath cycles, exhale, pulling your abdomen toward your spine and slowly roll back up; your head is the last to come up. If you feel flexible once in the forward bend position, try to alternate straightening one or both legs and then your back. Repeat the exercise 3 times.

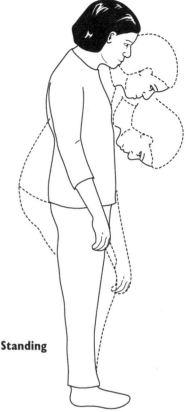

FIGURE 1.16 Standing forward bend.

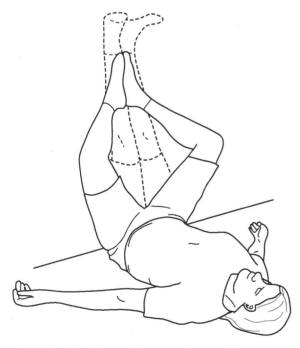

FIGURE 1.17 Elevated leg stretch on wall.

Elevated Leg Stretch on Wall

This exercise should be performed only before pregnancy, during the first trimester of pregnancy, or postpartum. Lie on your back with the soles of your feet together and your legs resting on a wall (figure 1.17). As you inhale, straighten your legs up the wall. As you exhale, pull abdomen toward your spine, bring the soles of the feet back together, bend the knees, and slide the feet down. Repeat the exercise 3 times.

Bound Angle

Sit in good posture with the soles of the feet together. Hold the ankles as your knees press toward the floor (figure 1.18). Stretch up through your spine. Lean forward and hold the position for 3 to 5 breaths.

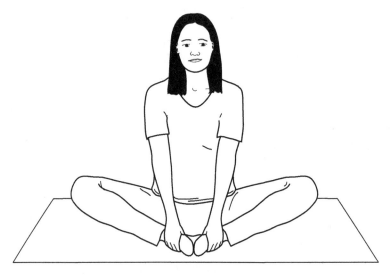

FIGURE 1.18   Bound angle.

Swan

From a tabletop position, move the right knee forward between the hands and extend the left leg back (figure 1.19). Use the abdominal muscles to stabilize the spine. Hold the position for 3 to 5 breaths. Exhale and move the right knee back. Repeat the stretch on the other side. If you are comfortable in this position, try to move the foot under the pelvis toward the side while opening up the angle of the knee.

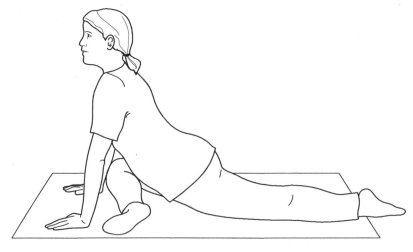

FIGURE 1.19   Swan.

Cooling Down

Many people think the cooling down part of exercise is a waste of time. However, the cool-down period is just as important as the warm-up if you want to decrease your risk of injury and restore balance in the body.

During exercise, muscle fibers, tendons, and ligaments are stressed. Also, waste products build up in the body. After exercise, the body needs to reestablish circulation, dissipate heat, and help muscles recover.

When you are exercising, your heart depends on your leg muscles to raise blood against gravity. When your leg muscles relax, veins fill up with blood. When muscles contract during exercise, they squeeze the veins and pump blood back up toward your heart. In this way, the alternating contraction and relaxation of leg muscles improves blood flow throughout the body as well as decreases the workload of the heart. This is especially important in pregnancy because the body's blood volume increases and circulation tends to become sluggish. When you stop exercising, your leg muscles stop pumping the blood against gravity and blood starts to accumulate again in the legs and ankles, a process referred to as *blood pooling*.

Blood pooling shifts blood flow away from the internal organs and puts additional stress on the heart. Less oxygen travels to the brain and also to the fetus. In pregnancy, this shift may cause women to feel faint or dizzy and even pass out. That is why the safety guidelines for exercising during pregnancy mention the importance of avoiding motionless standing for a long time. The cool-down period helps to reestablish circulation and prevent blood pooling and brings the oxygen and nutrients the muscles, tendons, and ligaments need to repair themselves.

There are four important parts to an effective cool-down. First, slow down aerobic exercise (walking, biking, swimming, and so on) to decrease your heart rate and breathing rate. Second, stretch the muscles, especially those worked during the exercise session. Third, rest the body with conscious breathing and relaxation. Finally, refuel your body with fluids and calories to help it repair itself and support the growing fetus.

Before ending your exercise session, slow down aerobic movements gradually. For example, if you were exercising by walking briskly, slow down the pace for about 5 minutes until you feel your heart rate and breathing slow down. In the Motherwell Maternity Fitness Plan, muscles are stretched throughout the exercise session. However, after exercising you should stretch any muscles that might still feel tight or sore or repeat stretches that felt especially good to you. Then lie in a comfortable position either on your back (only in the first trimester) or on your left side.

Close your eyes and try to relax your body. Concentrate on your breathing. Breathe deeply and slowly, imagining muscles releasing during each exhalation. This is also a good time to practice the breathing exercises described in chapter 3. Listening to soothing music will enhance your experience. Imagine your body is ice melting in the sun. Continue for about 5 to 10 minutes.

When you feel rested, roll onto your left side (or stay on your left side), and using your hands for support, slowly come to a sitting position. Take a couple more deep breaths and when you feel ready, slowly rise to a standing position. Once standing, walk around slowly to reestablish circulation. Be sure to replenish fluids immediately and eat a meal or snack within an hour after exercising.

Caring for Your Body During All Nine Months

Congratulations! You are going to have a baby. There is no other time in your life when your body goes through so many changes as in pregnancy. Practically every system is affected, including your mind, body, and spirit.

In our culture, women tend to obsess over their physical appearance through adolescence and early adulthood. Most women, however, know more about their clothes than the body they put them on. A recent survey in a national magazine reported that when asked, most young women say they are at least 10 pounds overweight, whether they are or not! One of the best things about being pregnant is not worrying about what you look like in a bathing suit!

As early as a few weeks after a woman becomes pregnant, she is alerted to changes occurring in her body. For some women, morning sickness is the first sign of pregnancy. For others, it might be the swelling of the breasts, the increase in hunger, or the skipped period. Some women find these changes to be unsettling. Others respond to the changes in their body during pregnancy with awe and curiosity.

Pregnancy provides a unique opportunity for you to see your body in a new light and to learn about the importance of focusing attention on the inside of yourself as well as on the outside. The changes that occur in your body during pregnancy will awaken you to the miracle that is happening in your body and in your life.

You may find that you appreciate your body in a different and exciting way. Most pregnant women become motivated to practice healthful behaviors to produce a healthy baby. However, it's just as important to continue practicing these behaviors after your baby is born. After all, who takes care of the caretaker? For the sake of both you and your family, you need to keep yourself healthy so you can function at your highest level. It's a well-known fact that when Mom is feeling good, everyone else around her will feel good too. The reverse also is true, or so you should have your family believe.

Getting Relief From Common Discomforts

Table 2.1 lists the 10 most common changes that occur in a woman's body during pregnancy, along with some of the resulting discomforts. Suggestions are offered for relief. There are many individual variations, so become aware of how your body responds to pregnancy. Notice daily, weekly, and monthly fluctuations in the way you feel. Try to view these discomforts as a wake-up call to pay closer attention to your body rather than as a nuisance, and you will experience pregnancy as a time of discovery.

TABLE 2.1   Common Changes and Discomforts During Pregnancy.

Common change	Common discomfort	Phase of pregnancy
The hormones of pregnancy tend to slow the digestive system.	Nausea and/or vomiting Heartburn Constipation and hemorrhoids	Usually first 20 weeks. Second and third trimesters Second and third trimesters
The cardiovascular system adapts to the increase in blood volume and the extra load on the heart. Blood vessels dilate.	Sluggish circulation Varicose veins Heart palpitations Low blood pressure Leg cramps Ankle swelling Headaches	Second and third trimesters Second and third trimesters Second and third trimesters Second and third trimesters Second and third trimesters Second and third trimesters Throughout pregnancy
Weight of breasts and enlarged uterus puts stress on the back muscles.	Lower back discomfort Upper back discomfort Nerve compression syndrome (carpal tunnel)	Second and third trimesters Second and third trimesters Second and third trimesters
Pressure of enlarged uterus relaxes pelvic floor muscles.	Urine leakage Increased risk for urinary tract infections	Second and third trimesters Second and third trimesters
Growing uterus puts pressure on the diaphragm.	Shortness of breath Rib cage discomfort	10 to 32 weeks Second and third trimesters
Hormones of pregnancy affect emotions.	Anxiety Depression Sleeplessness	You may notice symptoms even before you know you are pregnant. Symptoms can last throughout pregnancy and into the postpartum period.
Hormonal changes increase metabolism and internal core body temperature.	Less tolerance to heat*	Second and third trimesters
Increase in water retention.	Ankle swelling Nerve compression syndrome (carpal tunnel) Corneal changes, change in eye refraction	Second and third trimesters Second and third trimesters Second and third trimesters
Hormone *relaxin* secreted in the body. Relaxin softens cartilage in the pubic bone to allow for stretching; however, it affects all joints.	Risk of joint injury	Throughout pregnancy and up to three months postpartum
Increased appetite because of hormonal influences.	Excess weight gain	Usually most pronounced in first and second trimesters

*Women who are used to exercising prior to becoming pregnant may be able to cool their bodies more efficiently during pregnancy than women who were sedentary before becoming pregnant.

Digestive Problems

Nausea and *vomiting* are common during the first 20 weeks of pregnancy. To find relief, try various strategies to see what works best for you. Eating small, frequent meals helps prevent overdistending the stomach while providing much-needed nutrients. Sometimes nausea and vomiting occur more frequently in the morning. If this is the case for you, keep crackers by the bed and take a few bites before you get out of bed. Prenatal vitamins can also upset the stomach, so take them with your evening meal. Then, if the vitamins do upset your stomach, it will be while you sleep.

Sucking on ice cubes or an ice popsicle may numb the stomach. The same is true with cold sports drinks, which also help to replenish glucose and electrolytes if you also have a tendency to vomit. Sniffing or sucking on lemons may calm the stomach for some women. Wearing sea bands, commonly found in most drug stores, will also provide relief. Sea bands work by pressing on acupressure points on the wrists, helping relieve nausea and motion sickness. Instead of wearing sea bands, you can also press the area with a finger of the opposite hand (figure 2.1).

Some researchers believe that eating calcium-rich foods may also alleviate the nausea commonly felt during pregnancy. If you notice that you

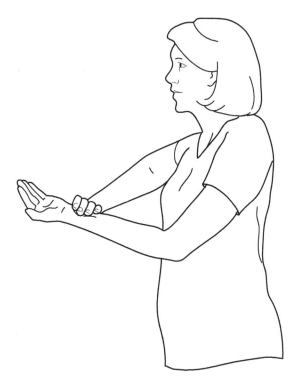

FIGURE 2.1 Pressing the acupressure point on the wrist with your fingers.

are not getting enough calcium in your diet and experiencing nausea, try drinking more milk or eating calcium-rich foods such as cheese, yogurt, or ice cream. Actually, the coldness of the ice cream may numb your stomach as well. If you have a hard time keeping food down, consult your health care provider.

Question: How do I find the pressure point that helps decrease nausea?

Answer: Place the first three fingers of your right hand on the inner aspect of your left wrist with the ring finger of the right hand directly over the wrist. Under the index finger will be the acupressure point. You can do this on either wrist.

In the early months of pregnancy, *heartburn* is caused by the relaxation of the lower esophageal sphincter because of an increase in the hormone progesterone. So each time your stomach contracts to push food forward out of the stomach, it goes backward into the esophagus, causing a burning sensation. Later in pregnancy, the increased size of the uterus presses on the stomach, also pushing food upward toward the esophagus.

Eating small, frequent meals may help prevent heartburn. Taking a short walk, staying upright after each meal, and sleeping with the head of the bed elevated allows gravity to help move the food in the right direction. However, if you are still experiencing discomfort, avoid spicy foods and high-fat meals to decrease the severity of heartburn.

During pregnancy, the increase in progesterone slows the digestive tract. This may result in *constipation* and, eventually, *hemorrhoids*. Drinking 8 to 10 glasses of water a day and eating high-fiber foods helps move food through the digestive tract more efficiently. Fruits, vegetables, and whole-grain foods provide additional fiber. Also, exercising stimulates the bowel. Try to walk after each meal. Avoid harsh laxatives and enemas. Seek medical advice if you experience severe pain.

If you avoid straining while trying to move your bowels, it will help reduce your risk of getting hemorrhoids. However, in the latter months of pregnancy the downward pressure of the uterus on the internal organs may also cause hemorrhoids. Hemorrhoids are a form of varicose veins, only in the rectum instead of in the legs. The most common symptoms are itching, bleeding, or pain around the anus. Hemorrhoids can be internal or external. Sometimes they need to be surgically removed, but usually they shrink and go away on their own.

To decrease discomfort from hemorrhoids, try to keep the anal area clean and dry and wash the area after each bowel movement. Warm soaks are soothing as are ice packs and hygienic pads. Avoid sitting for long periods on a hard surface and seek medical advice before using any over-the-counter remedies.

Sluggish Circulation

To alleviate sluggish circulation, avoid sitting for more than 20 minutes at a time and try to exercise at least 30 minutes on most days of the week. The pumping action of the muscles when you exercise or walk around stimulates circulation and helps to oxygenate the body.

Varicose veins are enlarged, twisted veins that can occur in any part of the body, but they are usually found in the lower extremities. In most cases, varicose veins are hereditary. However, you can reduce their severity through regular exercise. Special stockings are available through your health care provider if you need to stand on your feet for long periods or if you have chronic pain or discomfort. Also, avoid wearing restrictive clothing, especially around the knees and upper thighs, because tight clothing tends to further reduce circulation.

At no other time during a woman's life will her heart work so hard as during pregnancy. By the end of the second trimester, the heart rate increases 10 to 15 beats a minute and becomes very excitable. For this reason, it is not uncommon to feel *heart palpitations,* or a pounding sensation in the chest. Eventually the feeling passes, but in the meantime, most women react to palpitations by becoming more anxious, which in turn increases the palpitations. The best way to counteract this chain of events is to try to relax the body and slow the breath. See chapter 3 for various breathing exercises.

If palpitations persist, please seek medical advice. Even though heart palpitations are common during pregnancy, it is always a good idea to be sure that your heart is healthy and there is no other underlying problem.

The hormone progesterone relaxes the smooth muscle in the body to allow the uterus to expand during pregnancy. Unfortunately, it also affects the smooth muscle of the blood vessels. For this reason, blood pressure decreases. Most pregnant women become aware of having *low blood pressure* when they quickly rise from a sitting to a standing position. Gravity pools the blood toward the legs, shifting blood flow away from the brain, predisposing women to feeling light-headed or dizzy. To keep this from happening, slowly rise from a sitting or lying position and slowly walk around so the muscles of the legs can pump the blood back to the heart. If symptoms get worse, seek medical attention. Sometimes, pregnant women become anemic and also get this same sensation. It's always best to err on the side of caution.

Slowed circulation can also cause *leg cramps.* If you find you have leg cramps at night, place a pillow between your knees to improve circulation. Leg cramps can also be caused by a calcium deficiency. Be sure to consume adequate amounts of calcium in your diet or take a calcium supplement. Another cause of leg cramps is drinking too many carbonated beverages such as sodas. These beverages have phosphorus, and consuming too much of them can upset the calcium–phosphorus balance in the body, causing muscles to cramp. Vitamin C may help to prevent leg cramps. Again, try different things and see what works best for you.

When you feel a cramp coming on, flex the foot of the affected leg so the toes point toward your head. If this is difficult, ask your partner to do it for you. Avoid massaging the leg, however, because you can dislodge a blood clot if that is the cause of the cramp. If cramping persists or you notice redness on your calf that is hot to the touch, seek medical advice.

Swollen ankles are a common discomfort during pregnancy. Even brief periods of exercise help prevent pooling of blood around the ankles and feet, decrease swelling, and bring more blood flow to your baby. Swimming in water or soaking in a warm tub (not more than 90 degrees Fahrenheit) with water up to your neck will also improve circulation and reduce swelling in the ankles, hands, and feet.

Headaches during pregnancy are usually caused by poor circulation, dehydration, or sinus congestion. In addition to drinking 8 to 10 glasses of water a day, there are several techniques using pressure points that may offer relief.

For the head press (figure 2.2), close your eyes and place both thumbs behind your ears, spreading your fingers on top of your head. Make small circles with your thumbs and fingertips, slightly moving the scalp back and forth. Continue for about 10 to 20 seconds, stop for a few seconds to see how you feel, and continue further if desired.

For the temple press (figure 2.3), place two middle fingers of the right hand on the right side of your head at the temple and two middle fingers of the left hand on the left side of your head at the temple. Gently press both temples as you make small circles with your fingers. Continue for 10 to 20 seconds, rest, and then repeat if desired.

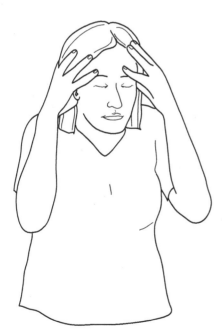

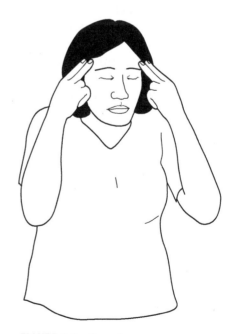

FIGURE 2.2   Head press.   **FIGURE 2.3   Temple press.**

For the eye relaxer, rub both hands together until you feel your palms getting warm. Close both eyes and gently place your warm palms over your eyes. Hold the position for 10 to 20 seconds and imagine the warmth from your hands spreading into your eyes and then spreading down into your body.

Stress is a common cause of headaches. In addition to the exercises just mentioned, practice the stress management techniques explained in chapter 6.

Muscular Aches and Pains

The pregnant body is changing inside and out. Structural changes create muscle tension especially in the back. To release tension, ask your partner to rub your back where it bothers you. There are also massage therapists who are specially trained to work with pregnant women. Ask well-meaning friends and family for gift certificates on your birthday, anniversary, or during the holidays. It will probably be the best gift you ever received! Massaging sore back muscles helps to relieve discomfort and is a great way to decrease stress. Studies of the general population show that the greatest cause of back pain is stress. In addition to massage, exercise (especially walking and stretching) is also an effective way to deal with muscle aches and discomfort.

Lower back discomfort. As the uterus becomes larger, it puts stress on the lower back muscles. Ideally, a woman strengthens her abdominal muscles before pregnancy and then maintains muscle tone throughout pregnancy. However, most women have weak abdominal muscles. The earlier in pregnancy a woman performs abdominal strengthening exercises, the less risk she has for lower back discomfort.

Walking and swimming are excellent exercises that relax the lower back and reduce discomfort. Sitting and standing with good posture also reduce excess strain. (See the good posture techniques later in this chapter.) When muscles in the backs of the legs are tight, they can pull on the back, creating more discomfort. Practice the stretching exercises for the legs and back in chapter 5. Resting in the knee–chest position (figure 2.4) will also help.

Upper back discomfort. The increased weight of the breasts along with the structural changes in the spine that occur during pregnancy cause rounding of the upper back and shoulders. Discomfort between the shoulder blades and across the back of the shoulders is common.

To relieve upper back discomfort, stretch the upper back frequently throughout the day (see chapter 5) and use good posture techniques. You can also place a tennis ball between your back and a wall and press your back against the ball wherever you feel discomfort.

Nerve compression syndrome, also known as *carpal tunnel,* is pain in the wrists that may radiate into the fingers. Some women also experience numbness and weakness, especially in the thumb of the affected hand.

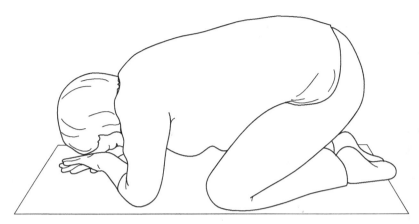

FIGURE 2.4   Knee–chest position.

The two most common causes during pregnancy are the increase in fluid retention and the impingement of the median nerve in the shoulder because of postural changes.

To prevent or ease discomfort, keep the shoulders in proper alignment, right below your ears. Also practice the shoulder stretches described in chapter 5. To stretch an aching hand, try this exercise. Extend the affected hand and grasp the fingers of that hand with your other hand. Gently pull the fingers downward until you feel a stretch along your inner wrist (figure 2.5).

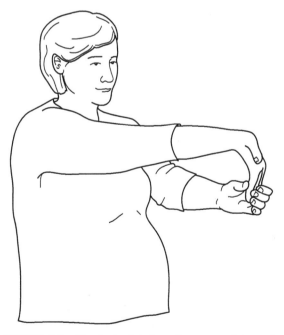

FIGURE 2.5   Hand stretch to relieve carpal tunnel.

Pelvic Concerns

Pressure of the enlarged uterus during pregnancy puts stress on the bladder and pelvic floor muscles. Usually by the second trimester, a woman starts to feel a sense of heaviness in her perineum. Oftentimes, this is accompanied by urinary incontinence (urine leakage) during coughing or sneezing as well as a sense of urgency when needing to urinate.

Pregnant women also are more prone to urinary tract infections than before pregnancy. When the uterus presses on the bladder, it impedes the woman's ability to empty her bladder fully, leaving a reservoir of urine to grow bacteria. Urinary tract infections are one of the most common causes of premature labor, so trying to avoid these infections is of utmost importance for you and your baby.

The best way to prevent or alleviate the leakage of urine when you cough, sneeze, or even laugh is to practice Kegel exercises at least 20 times a day as explained in chapter 1. In fact, the more Kegels you do, the better the results. If urine leakage continues despite your efforts, wear panty liners for comfort.

To prevent urinary tract infections, try to drink at least 10 glasses of water a day to flush out the bladder frequently. Drinking unsweetened cranberry juice helps by changing the acidity of the urine, making it an unfavorable environment for bacteria to grow. Also, try this exercise: When you urinate, pull your belly toward the spine to stimulate complete emptying of the bladder. Even if you don't have the urge to urinate, make a habit of emptying your bladder frequently throughout the day. If you have symptoms of an infection such as a burning sensation when you urinate, seek medical care to avoid developing a full-blown infection.

Breathing Rates

You may notice breathing changes as early at the first month of pregnancy. In early pregnancy, the hormone progesterone stimulates the respiratory center in the brain to take in more oxygen. This may give you a sense of getting short of breath. For some women, this is the first sign of being pregnant. Later in pregnancy, the uterus presses up on the diaphragm, restricting lung expansion and again, you may feel the inability to completely fill your lungs as you inhale.

Good posture while sitting and standing will give more space for your lungs to expand. Also, stretching the sides of the torso as described in chapter 5 will help you breathe more easily.

The upward pressure of the uterus also affects the rib cage. In pregnancy, the ribs tend to expand to accommodate this pressure. This expansion may cause discomfort. Try moving in different positions to alleviate discomfort, and practice good posture to create more room for the uterus. Practicing the belly breathing techniques described in chapter 3 may also provide relief.

The good news is that in the last few weeks of pregnancy, the baby drops and breathing becomes easier, so hang in there! While some shortness of breath is expected during pregnancy, severe symptoms may be an indication of a more serious problem. If you experience chest pain along with shortness of breath, seek medical care.

Emotional Challenges

The hormones of pregnancy affect women's emotions, the most common being anxiety. Physically, the body is changing day-to-day, creating fears about gaining too much weight and being able to continue pleasurable activities such as hiking, playing recreational sports, or even sex. Pregnancy can put a stress on body image, self-esteem, and marital relations.

Also, from the moment a woman discovers she is pregnant, she starts to worry about the fate of her baby. Common concerns include miscarriage, premature labor, gestational diabetes, or genetic diseases. There might also be personal issues such as finances, family dynamics, and career decisions.

Unresolved anxiety may result in depression and, more frequently, sleep disorders. It then becomes a vicious cycle: anxiety, sleep disorder, depression, anxiety, and so on. The following suggestions are ways to break this cycle of events and take charge of your emotional health.

Anxiety and depression. Getting a grip on anxiety is very basic: Only worry about those things that you can control. If you practice healthful behaviors during pregnancy, which you can control, then you are doing everything you can to promote a positive outcome. Exercising regularly, eating healthfully, and taking time to practice slow breathing as outlined in chapter 3 also will help reduce anxiety and prevent depression. Read more about stress management techniques in chapter 6. If despite all efforts you still feel depressed, seek medical advice.

Sleeplessness. In addition to anxiety disrupting your sleep, just finding a comfortable position during pregnancy can be a challenge. The most comfortable position for sleeping during pregnancy is lying on your side with your knees bent and pillows between your legs and behind your back.

Another reason many pregnant women have a hard time sleeping is the need to get up several times during the night to go to the bathroom. Avoid drinking large amounts of liquids after your evening meal and see whether this helps decrease the number of times you are awakened with a full bladder. Also at your evening meal, drink some milk. When milk is digested, an amino acid called tryptophan is produced, which helps induce sleep.

Insomnia may be a nuisance to you, but it will not hurt your baby. And who knows, maybe this is nature's way of preparing your body for sleepless nights after your baby is born!

Temperature Sensitivity

For some women, pregnancy is the only time in their lives that they are warm. This intolerance to heat is caused by the increase in metabolism that occurs during pregnancy. In fact, your internal body temperature rises during pregnancy as a result. You may also feel warmer from increased body weight and the work of carrying your baby around with you all day.

To relieve heat discomfort, layer clothing. Stay out of heat during the day and keep adequately hydrated. Take cool baths and avoid exercising to the point of profuse sweating. Intolerance to heat may continue into the postpartum period for a few months, especially if you are breastfeeding.

Water Retention

By the end of your pregnancy, you will have accumulated approximately 6 liters of additional fluid in your body. Fluid usually accumulates around your wrists and ankles. Frequently this is the cause of nerve compression syndrome (carpal tunnel), discussed previously in this section.

Women also need to be careful when performing sports with lateral movement such as tennis and racquetball. The increased fluid puts more stress on the ankle joint, predisposing you to injury.

In addition to the tips mentioned earlier to relieve ankle swelling, perform ankle circles throughout the day. Whenever possible, prop your feet up on a stool or chair. Read labels and try to avoid ingesting large amounts of sodium. Canned foods are prepared with probably more sodium than you need. There is also a belief that not eating enough protein during pregnancy will exacerbate swelling. Read about proper nutrition in chapter 4.

Water retention may also cause corneal changes or alterations in eye refraction. Wait to refract eyes until about 6 months after you deliver. Use glasses if contacts are no longer comfortable.

Joint Protection

The pregnancy hormone relaxin is responsible for softening the cartilage in the pubic bone to allow it to stretch during delivery. Unfortunately, it affects all the cartilage in the body, putting a pregnant woman at a greater risk of joint injury. To reduce the risk, avoid making quick changes in direction when walking or playing sports. Stretch the leg muscles daily to keep the muscles surrounding the knees and hips relaxed. Also avoid activities that encourage you to bounce at the knees. To reduce hip discomfort, perform exercises that strengthen your lower back and abdominal muscles, and take warm baths. The position of the baby may also press on areas of the hips. If so, change positions when uncomfortable.

Increase in Appetite

Nature protects the baby by making sure pregnant women are hungry. During pregnancy, though, you still should be mindful of what you are eating and in what amounts. Eat frequent, small, well-balanced meals, and avoid sweets and fatty foods. Follow the nutritional guidelines in chapter 4.

The average pregnant woman should gain 25 to 35 pounds. If you are underweight, you might want to gain more; if you are overweight, you might want to gain less. Refer to your health care provider for guidelines that suit you best.

Posturing for a Healthy Pregnancy

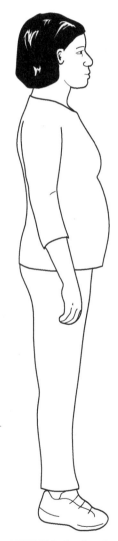

Proper posture can alleviate many of the muscular and skeletal discomforts of pregnancy as well as help improve mood. Attitude affects posture, and posture affects attitude. Think of a person who is sad or depressed. The head is usually slumped forward, the shoulders are rounded, and the abdomen protrudes outward. Think of a person who is happy. As she walks, she looks forward instead of downward, and she carries her body in anatomical alignment with her ears over her shoulders, her shoulders over her hips, her hips over her knees, and her knees over her ankles. The abdomen is pulled inward and upward, supporting the spine. There is even a lightness in her step. When you are feeling tired or sad, think about getting your body in proper alignment and notice how it makes you feel.

Pregnancy puts a tremendous strain on the back muscles. The curve in the upper back becomes more pronounced as the increasing weight of the breasts pulls the shoulders forward. The curve in the lumbar region of the lower back is accentuated because of the weight of the enlarged uterus. Be mindful of your posture and consciously correct yourself throughout the day.

Finding comfortable positions during pregnancy can be a challenge. Here are tips on recommended postures in several positions.

When standing, stand tall with your knees over your ankles, your hips over your knees, your shoulders over your hips, and your ears over your shoulders (figure 2.6). Imagine hugging your baby with

FIGURE 2.6   Good standing posture.

your abdomen by pulling the belly button toward the spine. Relax the buttocks and keep the knees soft (do not lock knees). Breathe deeply so that the sides and back of your torso, as well as your chest, expand when you inhale and relax when you exhale.

Rock forward and backward on the bottoms of your feet. Begin to make the movement smaller and smaller until you come to rest where it feels your weight is equally distributed between the front and back of your feet. Then, do the same thing while shifting your weight side to side. Slow the movement down and find where it feels your weight is equally distributed between both feet.

Get into the habit of positioning yourself into proper postural alignment in the morning and several times throughout the day. The more you practice standing in good posture, the more chance that standing in good postural alignment will become second nature to you.

When sitting, sit in a position that allows you to keep a slight inward curve in the lower back (figure 2.7). Keep the shoulders over the hips, and the ears over the shoulders. The knees should be bent at a 90-degree angle and either at or above hip level.

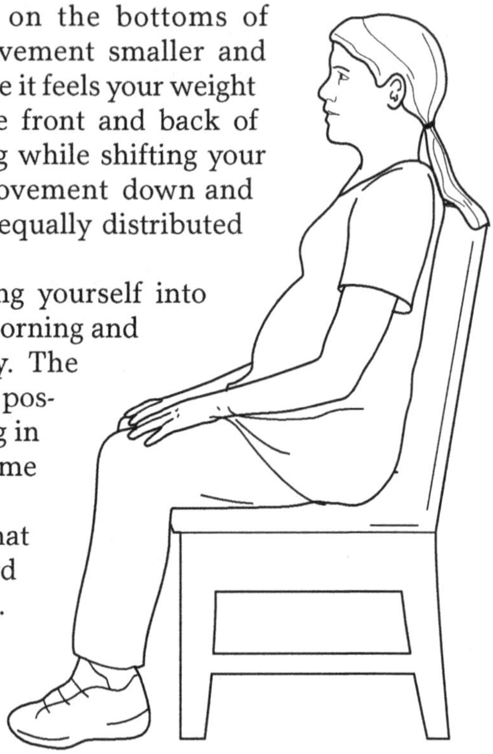

FIGURE 2.7 Good sitting posture.

When lying on one side, lie with the knees bent and the arms in a comfortable position. Place a pillow in front of your bottom leg and rest your top leg on top of the pillow (figure 2.8). The pillow can also be positioned between your knees. For added support, place a pillow in the small of the back as well.

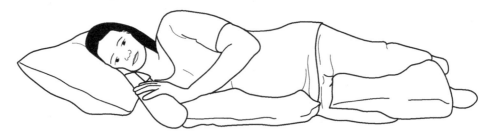

FIGURE 2.8 Good posture when lying on one side.

Protecting Your Back

In addition to your posture, how you move your body can affect comfort during pregnancy. Poor body mechanics can result in chronic back problems. Prevention is the key.

As your pregnancy progresses, you may find it hard to get up once you are lying down. Many people *jack-knife* to get up, meaning they sit up quickly by flexing at the hips. This maneuver puts excessive strain on the lower back. The most comfortable and recommended way to get up from a horizontal position is to bend your knees, roll onto your side, and then use your arms to push the body into a sitting position (figure 2.9).

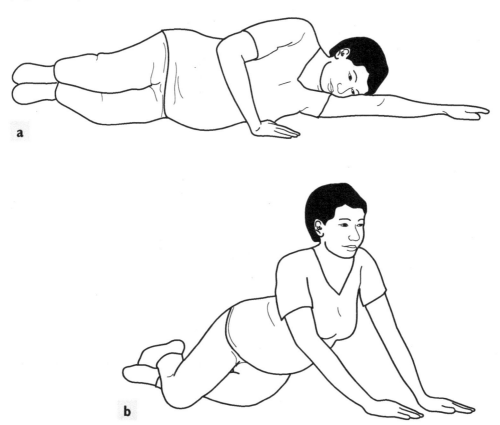

FIGURE 2.9   Getting up: (*a*) bend the knees and roll to one side; (*b*) use your hands to push to a sitting position.

Proper lifting is crucial to good back health. If you are having a healthy pregnancy with no complications and your health care provider says you can lift objects, please follow these safety guidelines to avoid back injury. Bring the object you are lifting as close to your body as possible. Bend at the knees and kneel down to pick up the object. Use your legs for strength as you stand up (figure 2.10). During the lift, pull the abdomen toward the spine for support. Take a deep breath and lift while exhaling. Do not hold your breath.

If you need to lift a small child, instruct him or her to stand on a chair or bench so you do not have to bend over.

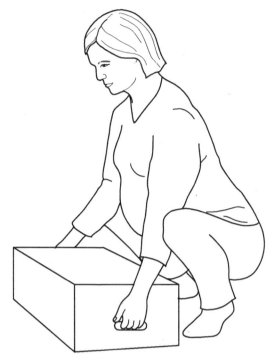

FIGURE 2.10   Proper lifting.

When you are pregnant, use your common sense about lifting large objects. If possible, ask someone to help you. Now is not the time to prove how strong you are!

Even housework can be made safe and fun. Vacuuming, sweeping, mopping, raking leaves, and shoveling snow are all activities that require long-levered tools. Use these activities as opportunities to strengthen leg, back, and abdominal muscles. By lunging forward and back in a diagonal fashion, you can turn household chores into beneficial exercises.

For the lunge, stand with one foot in front of the other and place your leg and foot slightly to the side. Bend the knee of the front leg and shift your weight forward (figure 2.11). The back leg remains straight. Shift your weight back while bending the back knee. Keep shifting weight back and forth while moving the tool and performing the task. This movement is more energy efficient than just using your arms and is less stressful for the back. If you really want to have fun, put on some music.

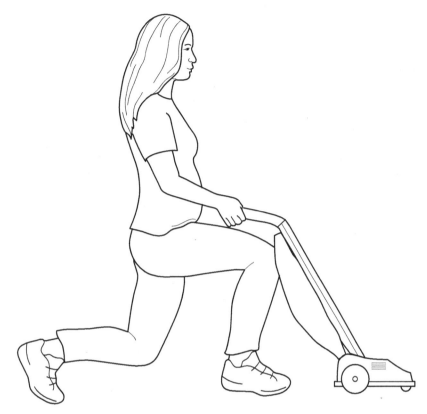

FIGURE 2.11   Performing the lunge while doing housework.

Going Easy on Your Feet

As pregnancy progresses, the feet tend to expand, sometimes in width, at least one size or more. Feet usually return to prepregnancy size along with the rest of the body after delivery. However, many women report that their feet stayed stretched. In any case, be sure to wear shoes that are the appropriate size.

A weight gain of 25 pounds or more increases pressure on the feet, which may add to the discomfort of existing bunions, blisters, calluses, hammer toes, ingrown nails, and heel pain. See a podiatrist if you have any of these problems.

Feet are often the most neglected parts of the body, and pregnancy is a great time to start paying more attention to them. Apply moisturizer to your feet every day to keep skin from cracking.

Regular toenail care is important. Cut toenails straight across when they begin to extend beyond the tip of the toe. Do not cut the corners. After cutting, file the nail smooth all the way around. When you can no longer reach your feet, consider getting a pedicure. Pedicures are a great way to care for your feet and relax at the same time. However, never put your feet in hot water. This may cause your feet to swell and blood pressure to lower. Soak your feet in tepid water instead.

For shoes, wear leather or breathable vinyl shoes with laces for adjustability. A ridged crepe or rubber sole will help with traction. Stick with flat heels for stability. Avoid clogs and high heels, which will add to your already unstable center of gravity. Avoid straps around the legs or ankles, which can restrict circulation. Rounded tips on your shoes for toe room is also advised. Feet move forward when walking and pushing toes into narrow tips is like putting a pencil into a sharpener—ouch!

Taking Care of Your Teeth

Almost 75 percent of all pregnant women develop *pregnancy gingivitis*. This is a swelling and bleeding of the gums that can lead to infection and discomfort. The prevention and treatment of pregnancy gingivitis is good mouth care.

Brush your teeth at least twice a day with a soft nylon brush. Brushing after every meal is ideal, but not always possible. Brushing before bed at night is most beneficial in getting rid of the sugar and bacteria that would ordinarily lie on the teeth all night.

See your dentist at least twice during your pregnancy for checkup and cleaning. Make your first appointment around the beginning of the second trimester when morning sickness is gone and you are still comfortable reclining in a dental chair. Routine dental Xrays should be delayed until after delivery. Consult with your obstetrical health care provider before allowing dental procedures other than cleaning to be done.

Caring for Your Breasts

The weight and size of your breasts increase during pregnancy. Sometimes, this increased weight can be uncomfortable and cause strain on the upper back and shoulders. For comfort, wear a supportive bra that pulls your breasts inward and upward.

Special care of the breasts during pregnancy is usually focused on preparing the breasts for breastfeeding. However, studies show that ointment, massages, and traction on the nipples are not always effective and may actually interfere with the breastfeeding process. Contact your local lactation consultant or nursing mothers group to learn more about preparing your breasts for breastfeeding.

After delivery, the nipples need to be kept clean and dry. If dried milk accumulates on the nipples, cleanse the areola (entire dark portion of the breast including the nipple) with plain water, especially before and after nursing. Also, continue to wear a supportive bra that does not constrict the breast. Avoid underwire bras; they may cause milk ducts to clog.

Throughout pregnancy and for the rest of your life, you need to practice a breast health program for the early detection of breast cancer. According to the Cancer Research Foundation, early detection and treatment of breast cancer saves lives. When detected early, almost 95 percent of breast cancer cases are successfully treated.

While you are pregnant, pick a day every month to examine your breasts. The first day of the month is easy to remember. Once your menses returns, examine your breasts 5 to 7 days after the first day of your period. Anything unusual should be reported to your health care provider. A complete breast self-exam includes checking your breasts in front of the mirror, while lying down, and in the shower.

Stand in front of a mirror with your arms at your sides and then reach over your head. Look carefully for changes in size, shape, and contour of the breast. Check for skin puckering, dimpling, or changes in skin texture.

While lying down, place a pillow or towel under your right side and put your right hand behind your head. With the three middle fingers of the left hand, examine all the breast tissue on your right side. This includes the area from your collarbone down to your bra line and from your armpit to your breastbone. Press your fingers into the breast using small, circular motions (figure 2.12). Repeat on the left side.

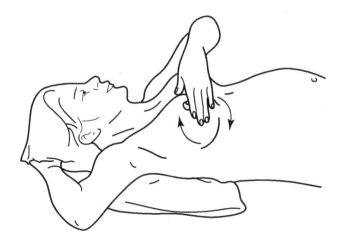

FIGURE 2.12   Breast self-exam while lying down.

While in the shower, stand with your right hand behind your head. Examine your right breast. With your left hand, use the examination techniques recommended while lying down. Then switch sides.

The combination of monthly breast self-exams, a yearly exam by a health professional, and a mammogram after age 40, has been shown to be the best way to detect breast cancer in the earliest stages. Regular exercise and healthful eating also will reduce your risk for cancer as well as other illnesses. If you need further instructions or have questions, discuss this with your health care provider. For more information, check out the American Cancer Society's Web site at www.cancer.org.

Caring for Your Skin

One of the most common skin changes during pregnancy is darkening. The exact cause is unknown, but it may be related to increased estrogen levels. In some women, darkening occurs on the face around the eyes. This is called *cholasma* or is more commonly referred to as the mask of pregnancy. Skin darkening will usually fade after delivery.

Skin darkening is made worse by exposure to the sun or other sources of ultraviolet light. Use sunblock with a skin protection factor (SPF) of at least 15 when you are outdoors, on cloudy as well as sunny days. Wearing a wide-brimmed hat will also help protect your face from the sun. There is some evidence that sun lamps and tanning beds may also promote skin cancer. Therefore, tanning parlors should be considered off-limits during and after pregnancy.

Moles may become more numerous during pregnancy. Most are usually not the type that can lead to cancer; however, it is always best to take precautions and check any suspicious moles with your health care provider.

The lifetime risk of melanoma, the most virulent form of skin cancer, is approximately 1 in 100 compared to 1 in 8 for breast cancer. However, because the cure rate for melanoma that has not spread is greater than 85 percent, the American Cancer Society suggests a monthly self-exam that can be combined with your monthly breast self-examination.

To examine your skin, stand naked in front of a full-length mirror near bright light. Begin by examining your scalp, then work your way down your body. Pay close attention to your lower legs, which is the most common place for melanoma to appear in women. To be thorough, examine your genitals, the inside of your mouth, and the backs of your ears. Use a partner or a hand mirror to examine your back. If you find a new mole or one that appears to have grown or changed color or looks different in any way, contact your health care provider.

Another common change in the skin during pregnancy is an itchy abdomen. As your skin stretches across the abdomen, the skin may become dry and itchy. The best relief is to use lotion or oil to moisturize the skin after bathing while the skin is still damp. If itching becomes intense, ask your health care provider about using an anti-itch cream with 0.5 percent hydrocortisone.

Spider veins, or vascular spiders, usually appear in pregnancy as a result of increased hormones. They look like tiny, red lines branching from the center, similar to spiders. They usually do not cause pain or discomfort, and they go away after pregnancy.

Numerous creams on the market claim to get rid of stretch marks around the abdomen, breasts, and hips. However, stretch marks develop deep underneath the skin in the connective tissue. Where you get stretch marks, or even if you get them, depends on your gene pool. If your mother had stretch marks, chances are you will too. There is nothing you can do to prevent them and nothing you can do to get rid of them. However, they eventually fade after delivery.

Question: Will the skin on my abdomen go back to the way it was before I was pregnant?

Answer: The skin around the abdomen stretches quite a bit during pregnancy. Imagine stretching a rubber band and holding it stretched for a long period of time. Typically, when you let go, the rubber band gets smaller, but rarely does it go back to its original size. Your skin acts the same way. Whether your skin stays somewhat stretched after your pregnancy is individual and really depends on your genetics.

Occasionally, pregnant women get itchy, reddish, raised patches on the skin called *pruritic urticarial papules* (PUPP). They usually start on the abdomen and spread to the arms and legs. It is not known what causes PUPP. Some suspect there is a genetic tie because it seems to run in families. Your health care provider can prescribe oral medications or anti-itching cream. Oatmeal baths may also provide relief. The rash goes away after delivery.

Other common skin changes during pregnancy include the following:

- Red and itchy palms; use moisturizing creams.
- Blotchy rashes on the legs that seem worse when exposed to cold.
- Skin tags that appear generally under the arms or breasts. They may go away after pregnancy or can be easily removed.
- Heat rashes; avoid hot baths and keep skin cool and dry.

Taking Time for You

Pregnancy is the only time in your life that you can sit on the couch and appear to be doing nothing, but really be accomplishing the greatest gift you have to offer, growing another human being. No matter what you do, you are being productive. So, don't feel guilty about resting when you are tired or just need some time to relax.

Try to schedule time each day to do activities you enjoy. In addition to exercising, plan to take a nap, take a bath, or just meet a friend for lunch. Ask other family members to help with daily chores. Remember, if you do not have your own plan, you are part of someone else's. Put yourself on the calendar first and then build your day around what *you* want to do!

Slow Dance

Have you ever watched kids on a merry-go-round,
    or listened to rain slapping the ground?
Ever followed a butterfly's erratic flight,
    or gazed at the sun fading into the night?
You better slow down, don't dance so fast,
    time is short, the music won't last.
Do you run through each day on the fly,
    when you ask "How are you?", do you hear the reply?
When the day is done, do you lie in your bed,
    with the next hundred chores running through your head?
You better slow down, don't dance so fast,
    time is short, the music won't last.
Ever told your child, we'll do it tomorrow,
    and in your haste, not see his sorrow?
Ever lost touch, let a friendship die,
    'cause you never had time to call and say hi?
You better slow down, don't dance so fast,
    time is short, the music won't last.
When you run so fast to get somewhere,
    you miss half the fun of getting there.
When you worry and hurry through your day,
    it is like an unopened gift thrown away.
Life isn't a race, so take it slower,
    hear the music before your song is over.

—*David L. Weatherford*

Your body needs a certain amount of down time to maintain a healthy immune system. Rest needs to take priority over cleaning the house, doing the laundry, or making the beds. If friends innocently offer to help you while you are pregnant, put them to work!

The superwoman myth is just that, a myth! Realize you do not have to prove anything. In fact, women who try to do it all are proving that they have a lot to learn. As in business, the intelligent boss is the one that surrounds herself with competent people. Empower friends and family and they will make you look very accomplished!

Spend time to live in the moment! Sit in a garden and listen to the birds. Breathe in the warmth of the sun on a sunny day. Pay attention to the sound the rain makes on the roof of your home. Around your birthday, anniversary, or holiday, ask for a cleaning service, or better yet, a gift certificate for a massage or whatever you find relaxing. Enjoy every moment of your pregnancy. Make every day special! You and your baby are worth it!

chapter | **3**

Breathing Routines for Two

Watch a sleeping baby. The baby's belly will rise and fall with each breath. Diaphragmatic breathing, or belly breathing, is natural and effortless. However, sometime in childhood we lose our relaxed belly breathing and start to breathe shallowly into the chest. Unfortunately, using shallow chest breathing for long periods creates tension in the body, limits the ability to take in oxygen, and causes fatigue.

> *We know that life begins with the first breath and ends with the last. But it is how we breathe in between the first and the last that greatly impacts how well we live this life.*
>
> **Nancy Zi**, *The Art of Breathing*

Understanding Belly Breathing

As you inhale, the diaphragm, the muscle that separates the abdominal and thoracic cavities, pushes down into the abdomen, causing it to protrude. Exhalation does the opposite, allowing the diaphragm to rise into the chest while relaxing the abdominal muscles. Research has shown that diaphragmatic breathing relaxes muscles, improves blood flow to the abdominal region, and calms the nervous system. It also helps tone the abdominal muscles and massages the internal organs.

The ideal way to breathe is in and out through the nose. The nose has tiny hairs that help clean the air as it enters the nasal passages. However, during pregnancy, nasal congestion is common. So, try to breathe in through your nose and out through your mouth. If this is still not possible for you, breathe in whatever way feels comfortable.

Question: How does diaphragmatic breathing help during labor and delivery?

Answer: Diaphragmatic breathing stimulates the parasympathetic nervous system, which calms the body. During labor, shallow breathing creates more discomfort, but diaphragmatic breathing helps to keep you relaxed. The more relaxed you are during labor and delivery, the less discomfort you will experience.

To make breathing effective, relax the jaw, tongue, and neck. Take a couple of deep breaths and focus on relaxing the tongue and jaw. You know your jaw is relaxed when your lips are parted slightly as you breathe. To relax the neck, perform this exercise: As you exhale, bring your chin toward your chest. As you inhale, bring head back on top of shoulders. As you exhale, bring right ear to right shoulder. As you inhale, lift head back up and repeat on other side. Repeat this one more time on each side or until your neck feels more relaxed. Be sure to breathe deeply and slowly.

Another way to relax your neck is to imagine you have a piece of chalk on the end of your nose. With your eyes closed, start to slowly draw figure eights on an imaginary blackboard in front of you, moving your head in one direction, then repeat the same motion in the opposite direction. Now you are ready to practice diaphragmatic breathing.

Old habits are hard to break, but here are five strategies to help you shift away from unhealthful breathing patterns to more relaxed diaphragmatic breathing.

1. *Learn to use belly breathing.* As mentioned previously, you are not really breathing into your belly. You are allowing the diaphragm to drop into the abdomen, creating more space for optimal oxygen intake. Belly breathing can be active or passive. In passive belly breathing, the belly expands during inhalation and relaxes during exhalation. This is the type of breathing that is ideal for relaxation and managing the discomfort of labor. In fact this is the breathing that is most commonly taught in childbirth education classes. Diaphragmatic breathing also is the type of breathing doctors recommend to people with asthma. When you practice relaxation belly breathing, your nervous system becomes calm and more air is able to enter the lungs.

Active belly breathing is used to strengthen the abdominal muscles, which support the spine while sitting and standing. Imagine breathing into the belly during inhalation while the belly expands and actively contracting or pulling in the belly during exhalation. Repeat this cycle a couple of times and feel the muscles of the abdomen being activated. After doing this a couple of times, you will also notice that the more forceful the exhalation, the deeper the inhalation. Here is an exercise for active belly breathing:

While sitting comfortably in a chair or on the floor, place both hands on your belly. Start with passive belly breathing. As you inhale, expand your belly, and notice how your hands rise away from your body. During exhalation, feel the belly relax and notice how your hands move back toward your body. Continue practicing a couple more times, then move into active belly breathing. Take a deep breath and expand the belly. As you exhale, imagine your navel reaching toward your spine. Repeat this sequence 10 to 20 times, focusing on expanding the abdomen during inhalation and actively contracting the abdomen during exhalation.

2. *Activate the muscles of the rib cage and back.* The lungs occupy space in the thoracic cavity, which is surrounded by the rib cage and spine. When passively belly breathing, in addition to using the muscles of the abdomen to induce diaphragmatic breathing, also think about relaxing the muscles of the rib cage and spine to breathe deeply.

Breathing is three-dimensional. Place your hands on both sides of your rib cage. As you inhale, feel the rib cage expand; as you exhale, feel the rib cage relax. Do this a couple of times. Then place your hands on your lower back. Notice that as you inhale, the back muscles expand and as you exhale, they contract. Now, relax your hands and take a couple of deep breaths, focusing on expanding and relaxing the entire upper torso. The following exercise lets you practice this breathing while in a different position.

Sit comfortably in child's pose (figure 3.1). Be aware of your breath as you inhale and exhale. Notice the rate and depth of your breath without changing it. Breathe into the belly while trying to keep the chest still. Now bring your awareness to the lower back. Notice how the back rises and expands as you inhale and contracts and falls as you exhale. Concentrate on releasing tension in the back with each inhalation. Next, observe how the muscles of the rib cage expand with inhalation and contract with exhalation. Try to relax your muscles to deepen the breath. Stay in this pose for about 5 breath cycles, observing all the movements and deepening your breaths.

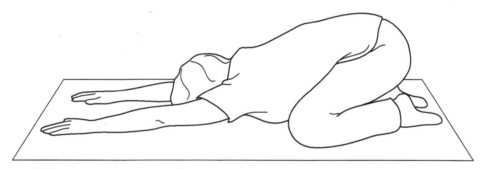

FIGURE 3.1   Become aware of your breathing while in child's pose.

3. *Reduce activity in the chest wall.* When the arms are raised above the head, the muscles of the chest are stretched and partially immobilized. Performing exercises that immobilize the chest wall will help develop awareness of diaphragmatic breathing.

Stand or kneel in good posture. As you inhale, raise your arms to the level of your shoulders and turn your palms up. Bring both arms above the head with the palms together (figure 3.2). Concentrate on lengthening through the rib cage and neck while pressing the shoulders down. Take 5 deep breaths, feeling the movement in the abdomen and lower sides of the rib cage. Relax the arms while exhaling and quietly notice your breath.

4. *Strengthen the diaphragm.* What you don't use, you lose. If you have not been belly breathing, then it's possible that your diaphragm is weak. The diaphragm is a skeletal muscle that can be toned and strengthened. The easiest way to strengthen the diaphragm is to consciously breathe deeply while performing exercises that offer some resistance to diaphragmatic breathing such as side bends and twists.

Stand with your feet 3 to 4 feet apart. Turn the right foot to the right at a 90-degree angle and the left foot to the right at a 45-degree angle. Turn the torso and hips forward. Keep both arms at shoulder level. As you inhale, raise the left arm and stretch it to the ceiling, palm turned in. During the next inhalation, reach the left arm over to the right as you bend the right knee and rest the right arm on the thigh (figure 3.3). Do not tilt forward or backward. Hold this position for 5 to 10 breaths. Consciously breathe into your left side and abdomen. Inhale as you return to center. Exhale and release both arms back to the sides. Notice how you feel. Repeat the exercise on the other side with the right arm. Perform the stretch twice on each side.

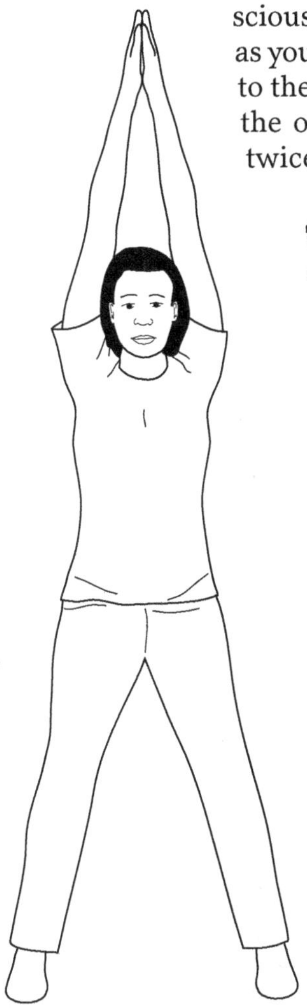

FIGURE 3.2   Raise the arms overhead with the palms together.

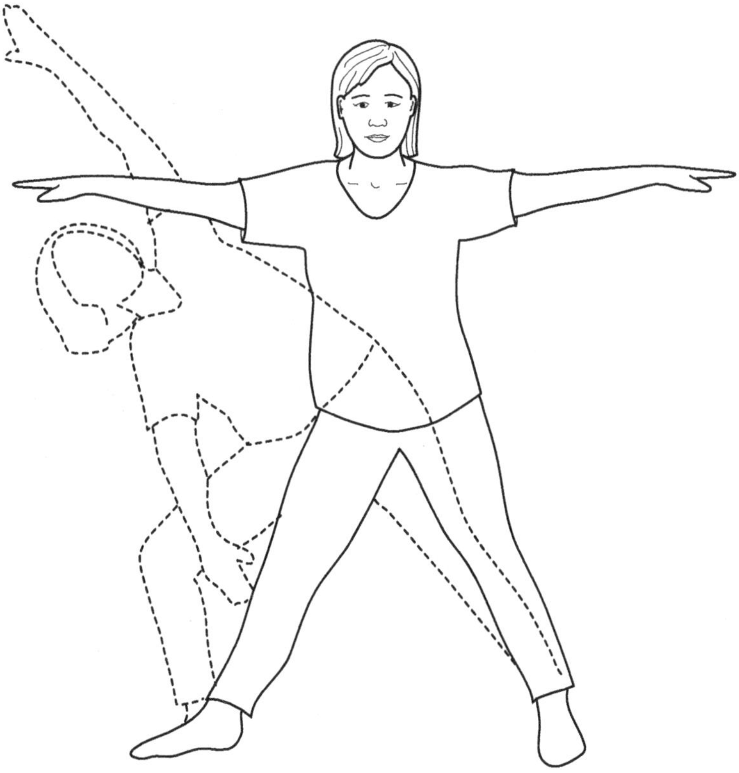

FIGURE 3.3   Side bends will strengthen the diaphragm.

This spinal twist pose also will help strengthen the diaphragm. Sit comfortably in a chair or on the floor. Extend your arms out to the sides and rotate the torso to one side. Stay in this position and breathe deeply using three-dimensional breathing for 3 to 5 breaths. Return to the center and relax. Repeat the twist to the opposite side. Perform this exercise again on each side and notice how you feel.

Breathe for good posture. Relaxation or belly breathing is great for reducing anxiety and preparing you for the labor and delivery experience, but when you are standing or sitting, your abdominal muscles should support the lower back. Sit or stand in good posture with your belly relaxed and notice how that affects your back. Now, pull the navel toward the spine and continue breathing while your rib cage and back muscles expand and contract. As you can see, this can be quite tiring if the muscles of your torso are weak.

However, the more you practice active belly breathing and three-dimensional breathing, the stronger your muscles will become. Every time you sit in a chair or have to stand in a line, practice good posture and try to keep your navel pressed toward the spine. At first, this seems unnatural, but practiced over time, you will notice your torso get stronger and belly breathing becoming second nature.

5. *Find your natural rhythm.* Just as everyone has a different fingerprint, breathing patterns are very individual. Sit quietly and just notice how you are breathing. Continue sitting comfortably, and start to concentrate on lifting up through the spine, releasing the shoulders into the back and lengthening the neck. Imagine a line of energy from the base of your spine through the top of your head, lifting you up toward the ceiling. As you inhale, notice the expansion on all sides of your body. Breathe diaphragmatically slowly and deeply, inhaling for two counts and exhaling for two counts. Take pauses between inhaling and exhaling and also between exhaling and inhaling. Continue this pattern for five breath cycles. If you are comfortable, increase your inhalation and exhalation to four or five counts. Be sure that the duration of the inhalation is the same as the exhalation. Find what feels right to you. Once you find the rhythm that is comfortable for you, stay with your breath and notice how deep, rhythmic diaphragmatic breathing makes you feel. Practice this breathing for 5 to 10 breath cycles.

Diaphragmatic breathing is calming for the mind and body. It also improves blood flow to the internal organs and tones and strengthens the abdominal muscles. The more you practice diaphragmatic breathing, the easier it will be to incorporate this breathing into your everyday life and reap the many benefits. This breathing technique will also help you during the labor and delivery experience.

Breathing Exercises

Unlike many of our bodily functions, breathing can be both conscious and subconscious. Most of the time, we do not think about breathing; it just comes naturally. However, the breath is a valuable tool for bringing balance into the body. The breath is the connection between body and mind.

In Oriental medicine, the breath is called *prana,* or life force. There is a belief that by practicing breathing exercises, a person is able to control the nervous system and eventually obtain control over the energy of the body as well as the mind. Yogis count life not by the number of years, but by the number of breaths.

When we consciously breathe, awareness of bodily sensations increases and we are able to communicate to the body with our breath. If we want to relax, we breathe slowly. If we want to become energized, we breathe quickly. If you want to relax a certain body part, think about breathing into certain muscles and see whether you can relax. The following exercises increase breathing awareness and will help you better utilize your breath for health and well-being.

Alternate Nostril Breathing

Alternate nostril breathing helps to aerate the sinuses and bring balance into both sides of the nose. As you improve airflow in the nostrils, you bring more oxygen to your body and to your baby. It also helps to focus the mind and enhances concentration.

Sit in a comfortable position with good posture. Close your right nostril with your right thumb (figure 3.4). Inhale through the left nostril. Close off the left nostril with your right pinkie finger, release your right thumb, and exhale through the right nostril. Continuing this breathing pattern for 5 breath cycles, then switch sides so that you inhale through the right nostril and exhale through the left. Be careful not to close both nostrils at the same time.

A variation of the exercise requires you to alternate sides with each breath cycle. Close off the right nostril and inhale and exhale through the left nostril. Then close off the

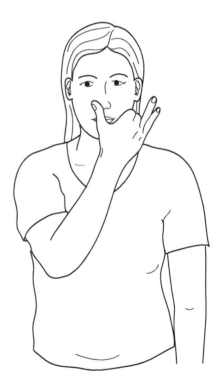

FIGURE 3.4 Alternate nostril breathing.

left nostril and inhale and exhale through the right nostril. Alternate sides for 5 breath cycles on each side.

The Water Pitcher (Three-Part Breathing)

Sit in a comfortable position and take some slow, deep breaths. Imagine your torso is a water pitcher. As you inhale, think about filling the pitcher from the bottom up, just as you breathe into the lower lobes of your lungs and then fill to the top. When you exhale, empty your lungs like a water pitcher, emptying from the top down.

When you inhale, you should notice your abdomen expanding first, then your rib cage on all sides, and then your chest. When you exhale, your chest will fall first, ribs will contract, and then your abdomen will pull in.

As you continue to breathe this way, you will notice that the more empty your lungs become, the deeper you will inhale. Continue breathing this way for 5 complete breaths and then sit quietly and notice how you feel.

The Eyedropper

This breathing exercise is similar to the water pitcher, except while exhaling, pull the navel toward your spine and empty your lungs from the bottom up instead of the top down. Try both exercises one right after the other and notice the difference in how you feel. Practicing this exercise will also help to strengthen the muscles of the abdomen.

Take a Breath!

Without breathing, life would cease to exist. Interestingly, babies practice breathing movements in utero even though they are not really taking any air into their lungs.

As you practice mindful breathing, imagine your baby practicing with you. As you inhale, visualize your baby inhaling at the same time. As you exhale, visualize your baby exhaling. This is a great way to connect with your baby before he or she is born and will bring you a sense of inner peace and contentment. Take a breath!

chapter 4

Eating for Fitness and Baby's Health

There are women who think that *eating for two* means eating twice as much. For some nutrients, such as protein, this is true. However, if you eat twice as much of everything, you will look like two even after you deliver. The key is to eat enough to support a healthy pregnancy, but be sure not to eat more than your body needs.

As mentioned in chapter 1, eating healthfully before pregnancy is ideal. However, regardless of how you ate before getting pregnant, there is no better time to adopt good eating habits than once you discover you are having a baby. Unfortunately, for the average woman in early pregnancy, nausea and sometimes vomiting will occur. So, getting good nutrition early on may be a challenge. Refer to chapter 2 for ideas on decreasing nausea. If you are vomiting excessively or are unable to keep food down, consult your obstetrical health care provider for other relief measures.

Gaining an Appropriate Amount of Weight

Gaining weight during pregnancy is a must for growing a healthy baby. The average full-term infant weighs between 6.5 and 9 pounds. General weight gain guidelines recommend that you gain 25 to 35 pounds during pregnancy. Typically, if you were underweight prior to pregnancy, your health care provider may suggest you gain more, and if you were overweight before you became pregnant, your provider may recommend that you gain less. Refer to your provider regarding how much weight gain is appropriate for you.

The preferred scenario is that you gain about 4 to 6 pounds the first trimester, 11 to 15 pounds the second trimester, and about 11 to 15 pounds the third trimester. The increased weight is distributed as follows:

Baby—6.5 to 9 pounds

Placenta—1.5 pounds

Amniotic fluid—2 pounds

Enlarged uterus—2.5 pounds

Enlarged breasts—3 pounds

Increased blood volume—3 to 4 pounds

Increased fluid—2 to 3 pounds

Fat stores and increased muscle—4 to 10 pounds

Total—24.5 to 35 pounds

So, get used to the fact that the scale will go up. How much you gain, however, can be controlled by proper eating and moderate amounts of exercise. The easiest way to monitor your eating is to count nutrients, not calories. Having said that, the rule of thumb, however, is to eat about 150 more calories per day in the first trimester and 350 more calories per day in the second trimester, according to the National Academy of Science. But if you follow the nutritional guidelines offered in this chapter, you will be consuming enough calories every day without eating excessively.

Develop a Sensible Eating Plan

In the 1960s, Lucille Ball became the first woman on television to sport her growing belly while pregnant. Her foods of choice were pickles and ice cream, and when she wanted it she had to have it or else!

To this day, husbands are shown in television shows and movies getting up in the middle of the night, driving through blizzards, jeopardizing their lives just to make their pregnant spouses happy! Most cravings are not that dramatic.

Some people believe that cravings are signals from your body that you need certain nutrients, but this has never been proven. While cravings are common during pregnancy, they are not harmful as long as you eat a well-balanced diet. Problems arise when a pregnant woman is satisfying her cravings with nonnutritive foods and then has no appetite to eat what she needs for herself and her growing fetus.

You need to have an eating plan not only to be assured you get proper nutrition, but also to avoid gaining excess weight. An eating plan ensures that you will get the foods you need, and then if you are still hungry, you can satisfy your cravings (within limit of course!). Having a plan also helps to reduce impulse eating. If you plan to bring a piece of fruit with you to the movies, chances are you will not be inclined to give in to the candy counter.

The definition of a meal is the portion of food taken at one time to satisfy the appetite. So, get rid of the idea of eating three meals a day. During pregnancy, it is important to consume nutrients throughout the day instead of trying to eat everything in two or three sittings. Ideally, you should eat at least 6 small meals a day: breakfast, midmorning snack, lunch, midafternoon snack, dinner, and evening snack. Bring your hands together with your palms open. The size of a small meal is what you can hold in both palms of your hands.

Your body is made to fuel and burn. It is much more efficient to eat only as much nourishment as you need to get you through the next several hours and then eat again. And because your blood sugar stays level this way, you have more energy for both you and your baby.

During pregnancy, you become more resistant to insulin, so most of the glucose in your bloodstream goes to your baby. Glucose is the only nutrient that fuels the growth of your baby. By eating small meals more often, you are constantly fueling your baby's growth. If, however, you go without eating for more than 4 hours, you risk becoming hypoglycemic (low blood sugar). The symptoms of hypoglycemia are light-headedness, dizziness, and nausea. Sometimes women even pass out or faint. Listen to your body. When you need to eat, choose food that gives you the best nutrients for you and your baby (figure 4.1).

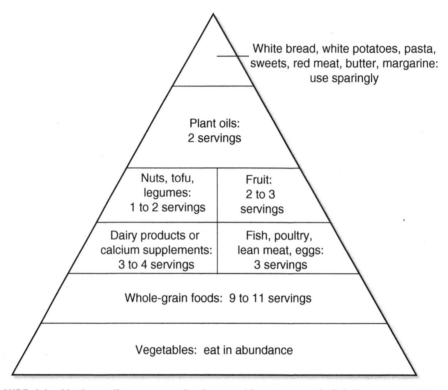

White bread, white potatoes, pasta, sweets, red meat, butter, margarine: use sparingly

Plant oils: 2 servings

Nuts, tofu, legumes: 1 to 2 servings

Fruit: 2 to 3 servings

Dairy products or calcium supplements: 3 to 4 servings

Fish, poultry, lean meat, eggs: 3 servings

Whole-grain foods: 9 to 11 servings

Vegetables: eat in abundance

FIGURE 4.1 Motherwell pregnancy food pyramid: recommended daily consumption.

Question: Some nutritionists now label foods that traditionally have been vegetables—such as corn, green beans, peas, and lima beans—as carbohydrates because of their starch content. Do you make these kinds of distinctions in your program?

Answer: While it is true that starchy vegetables should be avoided during a weight loss program, during pregnancy eating vegetables in general is a good thing. Whether the vegetables are more starchy than others really isn't an issue. The same is true with fruits, such as bananas, that typically have a higher sugar content. However, to obtain maximal nutrient benefit of all fruits without increasing sugar intake, eat fruit when ripe and avoid eating it when overripe.

Probably the hardest part of eating sensibly for most people is figuring out serving sizes. Table 4.1 lists different food groups and standard serving sizes for the most common foods in each group.

TABLE 4.1 Serving Sizes

Food group	Serving size
Dairy	1.5 ounces natural cheese 2 ounces processed cheese 1 cup skim milk, 1 percent or 2 percent milk
Fish, poultry, lean meat, eggs (protein)	3 to 4 ounces fish, poultry, or lean meat 1 medium egg
Nuts, legumes (protein)	1/4 cup nuts 1/2 cup dried beans or peas 2 tablespoons peanut butter
Fruit	1 medium piece of fruit 1/2 cup cooked or canned fruit 3/4 cup fruit juice
Whole grains	1 slice whole-grain bread 1/2 bagel or bun 1 ounce cold cereal 1/2 cup brown rice or whole-grain pasta

Keep a Food Diary

In the beginning, it might help to keep a food diary to keep track of what you are eating. Get a small notebook and record all of the foods or nutrients you eat each day. See the example in figure 4.2.

Keeping a food diary is an excellent tool for helping minimize excess weight gain. If you find you are gaining more than is recommended, look at your diary and see whether you are exceeding your number of servings or having more foods from the group at the top of the pyramid than you need. In reality, if you eat all of the required nutrients, you really do not need any foods from this group at all!

Use the 80/20 rule for eating nutritiously. As you eat throughout the day, make healthful decisions 80 percent of the time and eat what you crave 20 percent of the time. By eating this way, you will satisfy your cravings and might avoid bingeing.

Question: I usually exercise in the morning before I eat breakfast. Is that okay now that I am pregnant?

Answer: When you are pregnant it is very easy to become hypoglycemic (experience low blood sugar). That is why it is important to drink at least a glass of juice before morning exercise. Juice is quickly absorbed into the blood stream, will help keep your blood sugar stable, and usually does not cause stomach upset while you are exercising. Try drinking a noncitrus juice such as apple juice to avoid heartburn.

Date: *September 15*

Time	Food eaten	Amount	Food group/ nutrient	Cooking method
6:30 am	Whole-wheat toast with grape jelly	2 slices	Grains, fruit	Toasted
6:30 am	Egg	1	Protein	Scrambled in oil
6:30 am	Orange juice	8 oz.	Fruit	N/A
9:30 am	Plain yogurt with fresh strawberries	6 oz. yogurt 1 cup fruit	Fruit and dairy	N/A
12:30 pm	Chicken salad pita with olive oil dressing	4 oz chicken 1 pita	Protein, vegetable, grains, oil	Broiled chicken
3:30 pm	Peanut butter and whole grain crackers	1 serving pb 6 crackers	Protein, grains	N/A
3:30 pm	Milk	8 oz.	Dairy	N/A
6:30 pm	Whole-wheat pasta and tomato sauce	2 servings	Grains, vegetables	Pasta boiled
6:30 pm	Broccoli	2 servings	Vegetables	Steamed
6:30 pm	Salad and olive oil	2 servings	Vegetables, oil	N/A
8:00 pm	Low-fat ice cream	1 cup	Dairy, sugar	N/A
8:00 pm	Almonds	2 servings (1/2 cup)	Nuts (protein)	N/A

FIGURE 4.2 Sample food diary.

Get Your Vitamins and Minerals

Most researchers agree that if a pregnant woman eats a well-balanced diet, she probably does not need to take a supplement. However, studies show that taking a multivitamin early in pregnancy does help reduce birth defects. Also, even a well-balanced diet may not have enough of certain minerals such as calcium, iron, and folic acid. Therefore, pregnant women are advised to take prenatal vitamins and eat a well-balanced diet to be sure they are getting adequate essential nutrients.

One word of caution: Do not take more than one multivitamin a day. Some vitamins, such as vitamin A, are fat-soluble and can be toxic if ingested in large quantities. Table 4.2 lists the key nutrients you need during pregnancy as well as good food sources for getting them.

TABLE 4.2 Key Nutrients During Pregnancy

Nutrient	Recommended daily amount*	Function	Food sources
Protein	60 grams	Building block for baby's cells; helps make blood	Meat, eggs, legumes, nuts, fish, poultry, dairy products
Water	8 to 10 8-ounce glasses	Helps to build new tissue; carries nutrients and waste products in the body; aids digestion; helps chemical reactions; helps prevent premature labor; helps to create an adequate amount of amniotic fluid	Water, decaffeinated beverages, soups
Fiber	20 to 30 grams	Helps flush out the digestive tract; reduces constipation; helps rid the body of excess fat and cholesterol	Fruits, vegetables, whole-grain foods, legumes, nuts
Calcium	1,200 milligrams	Builds strong bones and teeth; helps muscle and nerve function	Milk and other dairy products, sardines and salmon with bones, collard, kale, mustard, spinach, turnip greens, fortified orange juice
Iron	30 milligrams	Helps develop red blood cells that bring oxygen to the baby; prevents maternal anemia and fatigue; increases immune function	Lean red meat, liver, dried beans, whole grains, enriched breads and cereals, prune juice, spinach, tofu
Zinc	15 milligrams	Helps produce insulin and certain enzymes	Meat, liver, seafood, milk, whole-grain cereals
Vitamin A	800 micrograms	Prevents eye disease; helps bones and teeth grow	Green leafy vegetables, deep yellow or orange vegetables such as sweet potatoes and carrots
Vitamin D	10 micrograms	Aids in utilization of calcium and phosphorus; promotes strong bones and teeth	Fortified milk, fish, liver oils, sunshine
Vitamin E	10 milligrams	Helps body use vitamin A; helps body develop red blood cells and muscles	Vegetable oils, whole-grain cereals, wheat germ, green leafy vegetables
Vitamin C	70 milligrams	Promotes healthy gums, teeth, and bones; helps body absorb iron; increases immune function; helps build collagen	Citrus fruit, strawberries, broccoli, tomatoes
Vitamin B_6	2.2 milligrams	Helps form red blood cells; helps protein metabolism and energy production	Beef liver, pork, ham, whole-grain cereals, bananas, vegetables
Folate (folic acid)	400 micrograms	Helps make blood; prevents neural tube defects and other problems; crucial to cell multiplication	Green leafy vegetables, dark yellow or orange fruits and vegetables, liver, legumes and nuts, fortified breads, cereals, rice, and pastas
Vitamin B_{12}	2.2 milligrams	Aids nervous system; helps form red blood cells	Animal foods, liver, milk, poultry; vegetarians may need to take a supplement

U.S. Food and Drug Administration (www.cfsan.fda.gov).
*Amount may vary depending on age, height, and weight. Check with your health-care provider.

10 Tips for Avoiding Excess Weight Gain

1. *Eat a good breakfast.* Skipping meals will contribute to eating in excess later in the day and may make you feel light-headed around midmorning. Also, after you sleep 6 to 8 hours a night without eating, your baby needs the calories early in the day. There is a theory that pregnant women should wake up at night to eat. I don't believe this is necessary, but try to eat a nutritious breakfast.

2. *Plan meals.* Think about what you will eat for most meals in the morning so you can budget your nutrients. Take healthful snacks such as carrot sticks, fruit, and whole-grain crackers to work. Without planning, you open yourself to whatever entices you through the day.

3. *Choose foods both low in fat and sugar and high in fiber.* Canned fruits, for instance, are usually packed in syrup. Read labels for fat and sugar content, especially salad dressings. If you choose to eat something with a high sugar content, also try to eat something nutritious such as a glass of milk. This may help prevent a spike in blood sugar that often stimulates fat storage to occur. Also, it is very common to feel hungry 20 minutes after eating a sugary food because sugar stimulates production of insulin. Fiber tends to make you feel fuller and aids in excess fat removal.

4. *Broil, bake, or steam your foods.* Even when you go a restaurant, ask about how your food is prepared. Most restaurants will accommodate your dietary needs.

5. *Go shopping for food on a full stomach.* Make a shopping list to resist impulse buying.

6. *Eat before you go to a party or social gathering.* The fuller you are when you arrive, the less chance you will be tempted to eat something you do not want.

7. *Smuggle fruit into the movies.* I can assure you that anything you buy at the movie theater is probably high in fat, sugar, or both. Plan ahead and you will save money as well.

8. *Drink at least 8 glasses of water a day.* Dehydration often is misinterpreted as hunger. If you are eating all of your nutrients and are still hungry, you might need to drink more water.

9. *Avoid people who want you to overeat!* People love to encourage pregnant women to eat everything they themselves want but know they should not eat. It is human nature. Do not eat to please anyone. You can still be polite. Just say, thanks, but no thanks!

10. *Eat mindfully and savor every bite!* Studies show that when a person eats with other people, there is a tendency to eat almost 750 calories more than when eating alone. Researchers attribute this to eating without thinking about what you are eating. Try this eating meditation: Take a bite of food and chew 50 times before swallowing. Notice how the food tastes and then notice how full you feel from just one bite. The more slowly you eat, the less food you will tend to consume and you will enjoy your food more.

Nutritional Considerations for Vegetarians

Eating patterns for vegetarians vary considerably. The lacto-ovo vegetarian eats grains, vegetables, fruits, legumes, seeds, nuts, dairy products, and eggs. The vegan diet includes all of these foods with the exception of eggs, dairy, and any other products coming from animals.

Studies indicate that vegetarians often have lower morbidity and mortality rates than nonvegetarians. Birth weights of infants born to well-nourished vegetarian women have been shown to be similar to birth-weight norms and to birth weights of infants of nonvegetarians. However, dietary deficiencies have been observed in very restrictive diets, so a well-planned vegan or lacto-ovo vegetarian diet will assure adequate nutrients for both mother and baby.

In pregnancy, protein and calcium needs double. For the lacto-ovo vegetarian pregnant woman, eating more eggs and milk products will assure adequate amounts of both protein and calcium. According to the American Dietetic Association, protein plant sources alone can provide adequate amounts of essential amino acids as long as a variety of plant foods are eaten and energy needs are met. Plant foods high in calcium include legumes, soy, almonds, collard greens, broccoli, calcium-fortified orange juice, figs, and blackstrap molasses.

The vegan pregnant woman should ingest more plant protein sources such as legumes, nuts, and soy. Pregnant and lactating vegans also should supplement with 2.0 micrograms and 2.6 micrograms, respectively, of vitamin B_{12} daily. If sun exposure is limited, they should supplement with 10 micrograms of vitamin D daily. Folic acid supplementation is recommended for all pregnant women, although vegetarians typically have higher intakes of folic acid through their diets than nonvegetarians.

When planning vegetarian meals (figure 4.3), choose a variety of foods, including whole grains, vegetables, fruits, legumes, nuts, seeds, soy, and, if desired, eggs and dairy products. If excess weight gain is a concern, choose low-fat dairy. Choose whole, unrefined foods and minimize the intake of sweets, fats, and highly refined foods. Eat a variety of fruits and vegetables and drink lots of water. Add nuts, legumes, and leafy green vegetables to soups and casseroles.

Breast-fed infants of vegetarian mothers should be given iron supplements at 4 to 6 months of age. If sun exposure is limited, these infants should be given a source of vitamin D. Breast-fed infants of vegan mothers should receive vitamin B_{12} supplements if the mother's diet is not fortified.

The need for iron also increases during pregnancy, especially in the later stages. Good vegetarian sources of iron include whole-grain cereals, green vegetables, and dried fruits. Iron absorption will increase if iron-rich foods are eaten with vitamin C, which is found in fresh fruits and vegetables.

Breakfast:	*Orange juice*
	Toasted whole-wheat bagel with jam
	2 scrambled eggs
	Decaf coffee or tea
Midmorning snack:	*Yogurt with fruit*
Lunch:	*Veggie burger with melted cheese on top*
	Whole-wheat bun
	Lettuce and tomato
	Carrots and celery with olive oil vinaigrette
	Fruit
	Water or decaf beverage
Midafternoon snack:	*Crackers with peanut butter*
Dinner:	*Stir-fry vegetables with steamed tofu cooked in olive oil*
	Brown rice
	Decaf beverage
Late night snack:	*Handful of almonds or walnuts*

FIGURE 4.3 Sample menu for a pregnant vegetarian.

Foods to Avoid During Pregnancy

Seafood is a naturally low-fat source of protein and an important part of a balanced diet during pregnancy. Fish also is a great source of omega-3 fatty acids, which are essential to a healthy body. However, according to the U.S. Food and Drug Administration, certain types of seafood contain enough methylmercury to cause damage to the fetus's nervous system.

The National Academy of Sciences estimates that up to 60,000 children are born in the United States each year with neurological problems thought to be caused by methylmercury exposure in utero. Nearly all fish contain trace amounts of methylmercury, but longer-living, larger fish that feed on smaller fish pose the largest threat to pregnant women. The fish most likely to have the highest levels of methylmercury include shark, swordfish, king mackerel, and tilefish.

The FDA advises to eat less than 12 ounces per week of cooked fish. They recommend shellfish, canned fish, smaller ocean fish, or farm-raised fish. The Environmental Protection Agency suggests that pregnant women, nursing mothers, and young children eat only one meal per week of fresh-water fish caught by family members or friends.

Another concern of eating seafood during pregnancy is the risk of parasitic infection. This is most common in uncleaned, raw, or undercooked fish. When buying fish and shellfish, look for the Grade A label and the U.S. Department of the Interior shield. Look for fish that are shiny with unfaded skin, red gills, and clear eyes. A mild odor is okay. Frozen fish should be in airtight packaging and solidly frozen. When you purchase fish, refrigerate it immediately and cook it within the next 48 hours. Freeze the fish if you are not going to eat it within the next three days. Fish can stay in the freezer safely for three to six months.

Fish is not the only food to be concerned about. Chicken and beef can also harbor harmful parasites and bacteria. Wash your hands before and after handling any raw foods. Cook meats thoroughly and carefully clean all surfaces the raw food touched. Pregnant women also are advised to avoid soft cheeses such as Brie because of the risk of listeria. Eat cottage cheese or hard cheeses instead. Even free-range eggs have been found to contain salmonella, so you should avoid raw or lightly cooked eggs.

chapter 5

Stretching and Strengthening Your Pregnant Body

Only 100 years ago, medical doctors believed that physical exercise and women's health were incompatible. At the end of the 19th century, physicians believed that female organs would "slip" and fertility would be impaired if a woman participated in sports.

The 20th century saw major changes in attitudes regarding women and sports. By the mid-1900s, women were finally allowed to compete in the Olympics. But it wasn't until 1984 that women were first allowed to compete in marathons.

Now, we have pregnant women running marathons. Ingrid Christiansen, a Norwegian long-distance runner, competed until her fifth month of pregnancy and delivered a healthy baby boy without complications. Competing in marathons is not something routinely recommended for pregnant women. However, research supports the belief that moderate exercise is safe in pregnancy and offers many benefits, including the following:

- Prevention or reduction of most pregnancy-related symptoms including back pain, ankle swelling, fatigue, venous thrombosis, and varicose veins
- Enhanced psychological well-being
- Reduced cardiovascular stress
- Reduced incidence of preeclampsia
- Prevention of excess weight gain
- Maintenance of fitness
- Easier labor and delivery
- Faster recovery after delivery

Swimming is especially beneficial during pregnancy. Because of the water's inherent buoyancy, water fitness classes offer less stress on the joints than weight-bearing exercise on land. Due to the hydrostatic pressure of water, extravascular fluid is pushed into the intravascular space, reducing edema, which is a frequent source of discomfort during pregnancy. Exercising in water also reduces heart rate and offers thermoregulatory advantages compared to exercising on land.

There is controversy about the effects of exercise on the length and type of delivery. Evidence suggests, however, that higher levels of fitness and activity may lead to shorter periods of labor. There is consensus that strengthened abdominal and pelvic muscles as well as a positive attitude toward labor enhance the probability of a vaginal delivery versus a cesarean section. Studies have also found a significant reduction in the perception of pain during labor in women who exercised during pregnancy.

Maternal Responses to Exercise

There is much concern about weight gain during pregnancy. Exercise can be safely performed throughout pregnancy provided the woman is in good health and exercise intensity is kept at a moderate level.

Studies show that pre- and postnatal women who perform weight-bearing exercise at 50 percent or more of their prepregnancy levels tend to gain less weight, deposit and retain less fat, feel better about their bodies, have shorter, less complicated labors, and recover more rapidly than women who either stop exercise or don't exercise at all.

In addition to exercise, eating nutritiously is an important part of the equation in assuring a healthy pregnancy. Pregnant women need to eat adequately and regularly to ensure that the baby is getting enough glucose to sustain growth. *Remember, moderate exercise + nutritious eating = healthy pregnancy.*

The benefits of exercise during pregnancy are additive. The ideal situation is the woman who is fit before pregnancy and then maintains fitness during pregnancy. However, even the unfit woman reaps many benefits of exercising while pregnant. It is important that both groups of women listen to their bodies and exercise at intensities that feel right to them.

Improved Cardiovascular Health

The cardiovascular changes that occur in pregnancy are very similar to those induced by exercise. Both increase blood volume, maximal cardiac output, blood vessel growth, the ability to dissipate heat, and the delivery of oxygen and nutrients to the tissues. For this reason, researchers believe that fit women have an easier time adapting to the physiologic changes of pregnancy than unfit pregnant women. This is why it is ideal to exercise and attain healthful fitness levels before getting pregnant.

One difference between the cardiovascular effects of exercise and pregnancy, however, is where the blood goes. With exercise, the blood flow is routed to the heart, skin, muscles and adrenal glands. In pregnancy, more blood is directed to the reproductive organs, kidneys, and skin.

Although the combined effects of exercise and pregnancy are additive, from a safety standpoint, there is concern that exercising too vigorously during pregnancy will shunt blood away from the internal organs and the fetus to the working muscles and skin, resulting in less blood flow to the baby. While fit pregnant women may have less blood shunting than unfit women, research shows that mild to moderate exercise is best for the pregnant woman.

Fit or unfit, women notice the benefits of exercise almost immediately. Moderate exercise improves sluggish circulation, reduces extravascular fluids that result in ankle swelling and nerve compression syndrome, prevents and alleviates leg cramps, and increases energy levels.

Improved Stamina and More Energy

Regular, sustained exercise increases the oxygen-carrying capacity of hemoglobin so that with each breath, more oxygen is delivered to the tissues as well as the growing fetus. This puts less strain on the heart muscle and contributes to increased stamina. Exercise also increases the number of mitochondria in the muscle cells, which helps to increase energy production, strength, and muscular endurance.

It is a puzzle whether high-energy women exercise or exercising women have more energy. In any case, women who exercise throughout pregnancy seem to be more organized, accomplish more tasks, and feel more energetic than sedentary women.

Pregnancy in itself is an aerobic workout. Just by virtue of being pregnant, a woman's body is overloading every day! The combination of exercise and pregnancy improves maximal aerobic capacity even more. Athletic trainers have noticed this for many years. They have seen female athletes dramatically improve their performance in national and international track and field events after having a baby. In the 1950s, several European trainers encouraged their female athletes to get pregnant to compete more successfully.

With increased oxygen demands, the fit pregnant woman is much more effective in delivering oxygen to her baby. From a safety factor, however, too much exercise could theoretically compete with the baby for oxygen. Therefore, it is important that women listen to their bodies when exercising. If you find it difficult to talk while exercising, then the intensity level is too high. Using a rating of perceived exertion for measuring exercise intensity is extremely important and a much better indicator of intensity than taking the heart rate in pregnancy. Also, by the time a woman stops to take her pulse, her heart rate has probably already dropped.

Rating of perceived exertion allows you to estimate your level of exercise intensity based on physical sensations such as muscle soreness, fatigue, and ability to breathe. The model rates perceived exertion on a scale of 1 to 10, with 1 being the least intense and 10 being maximal intensity. As you exercise, choose a number between 1 and 10 that approximates your level of exertion. Use a combination of all sensations, not just one. Plan to exercise in the 5 to 8 range at least 30 minutes every day.

Enhanced Ability to Handle Heat Stress

Regular exercise over a sustained period tends to increase blood volume to the skin, which helps to dissipate heat. Exercise also decreases the core temperature threshold for perspiring. With exercise, over time the body becomes extremely efficient at keeping the body cool.

In pregnancy, the body's set point for normal body temperature decreases as the internal body temperature increases 0.5 degrees centigrade. This, in combination with the increased blood flow to the skin, helps pregnant women keep their bodies cool.

So, the effects of pregnancy and exercise are additive. That is why a pregnant woman who exercises regularly can deal more effectively with heat stress than a sedentary pregnant woman.

Increased Metabolic Capacity and Insulin Sensitivity

Pregnancy is an anabolic process. Every day, the pregnant woman is growing new tissue. To support this tissue growth, the metabolic rate increases by about 15 to 20 percent at rest. The metabolic system also increases insulin resistance to keep glucose levels high for fueling the baby's growth. In this way, the pregnant woman utilizes energy similar to a diabetic.

Exercise increases metabolic capacity by increasing muscle mass and training the body to use fat stores to supply energy. Regular exercise also increases insulin sensitivity, resulting in more glucose utilization by the maternal cells. Researchers studying the effects of exercise in diabetes have found that regular exercise frequently reduces the need for insulin. This might also be the case for gestational diabetics. More studies need to be done.

In general, the combined effect of exercise and pregnancy increases the use of fat for energy and improves supply of glucose to the baby, provided the pregnant woman eats adequately and regularly. Small, frequent meals and moderate exercise help to sustain a healthful level of blood sugar and contribute to a healthy pregnancy for both mom and baby.

Improved Musculoskeletal Function

The stronger and more fit a woman is before getting pregnant, the fewer problems she has in adjusting to the musculoskeletal demands of pregnancy. Pregnant women with strong abdominal and back muscles tend to have a lower incidence of lower-back discomfort throughout pregnancy. During pregnancy, the hormone relaxin causes increased joint laxity, creating more instability. Having strong joints reduces the risk of injury.

There is a question of whether a stretched muscle can be strengthened. For this reason, it is important for women to work on strengthening their abdominal muscles early in pregnancy.

More stress is also placed on the upper back from the normal increased curve of the spine as well as the increased size and weight of the breasts. Exercises that concentrate on strengthening the upper back and stretching the chest muscles help to counteract any discomfort that may occur.

Decreased Maternal Discomforts

Researchers found that women who continued to perform weight-bearing exercise during pregnancy gained less weight and accumulated less fat than their sedentary counterparts while staying within the normal weight gain guidelines for pregnancy.

They also discovered that women who are fit before pregnancy have an easier time preventing fat disposition and excessive weight gain with exercise than unfit women. Women who exercise regularly tend to burn more calories than unfit women exercising at the same intensity. However, in both groups, it is recommended to exercise moderately 20 to 40 minutes on most days of the week to limit weight gain and fat disposition.

Studies indicate that women who exercise regularly during pregnancy have less than 10 percent occurrence of lower back, leg, or pelvic discomfort compared to nonexercisers, who reported more than a 40 percent incidence. The three factors that seem to influence a decrease in maternal discomforts include exercise that is regular, weight-bearing, and sustained over time. There is also evidence that regular physical activity during the year before pregnancy and during early pregnancy reduces risk of preeclampsia, which can be a life-threatening situation for both mother and baby.

Regular exercise in the general population is associated with a lower incidence of upper respiratory infections. Researchers have observed that exercising pregnant women experience a lower incidence of colds, flu syndromes, sinusitis, and bronchitis. On the other end, people who exercise too strenuously have an increased incidence of upper respiratory infections. Moderation is the key to health!

Easier Labor and Delivery

Research suggests that women who continue regular weight-bearing exercise throughout pregnancy show a marked decrease in the need for pain relief during labor, in the incidence of maternal exhaustion, and in the need for artificially rupturing the membranes to stimulate the progression of labor.

These women also have a lower incidence of induced labors, episiotomies, abnormal fetal heart rates, and the need for operative interventions such as forceps and cesareans. Researchers also find a significant reduction in the overall duration of labor in women who continue to exercise throughout pregnancy.

Positive Attitude

Pregnant women and new mothers who exercise tend to have a more positive attitude than those who don't. The question is whether the positive attitude motivates the woman to exercise or the exercise causes a positive attitude. In any case, women who exercise regularly during and after pregnancy report a better body image and overall feeling of wellness.

Physiological Considerations

Despite the many advantages of exercise during pregnancy, there are still concerns about exercising at high intensities. Historically, pregnant women have been advised to continue activities that were practiced before pregnancy and not to start anything new. That was adequate advice when women did not participate in sports. However, now many women are lifting weights, kickboxing, and attending Spinning classes, and want to continue after becoming pregnant. The problem is that these activities tend to be high in intensity and may not be suitable for expectant moms.

Also, researchers have noticed that women who begin performing mild- to moderate-intensity exercises during pregnancy gain many health benefits if properly supervised. At no other time in a woman's life is her body as stressed as it is in pregnancy. Practically every organ system and muscle group is affected by pregnancy.

However, every pregnant woman is different in her response to exercise, depending on her health and fitness level before pregnancy. For this reason, exercising expectant moms need to listen to their bodies and modify exercise when appropriate. The American College of Obstetricians and Gynecologists (ACOG) guidelines advise that pregnant women stop exercising when fatigued and not exercise to exhaustion.

Question: I have been taking Spinning classes for several years. Can I continue to take classes now that I am pregnant?

Answer: The intensity of Spinning classes may be too high, depending on the level of resistance you choose as well as the amount of time you spend on the bike in one session. So, while I would not recommend starting a Spinning class during pregnancy, if you are already used to Spinning and want to continue, here are some safety measures to reduce your risk of injury:

1. Stay well-hydrated.
2. Spin no more than 30 minutes in a session.
3. Lower the resistance to lower the intensity. Be sure you can talk while you are exercising.
4. Listen to your body. Slow down when you get tired and stop when you feel fatigued.
5. If you feel any discomfort in your knees, stop Spinning while you are pregnant and walk or swim instead. Knees are more vulnerable to injury during pregnancy.
6. Eat an adequate number of calories to offset calories burned during exercise.
7. Consult your health care provider.

Body image is a concern for all pregnant women, but especially for those women who regularly exercised to attain optimal body proportions before pregnancy. During pregnancy, exercise goals need to change to assure a healthy pregnancy. The enlarged belly and increased fat deposits on the hips and thighs are necessary adaptations for fetal development and protection.

A positive attitude toward these physical changes allows the pregnant woman to modify exercise appropriately and enjoy this very special time in her life. The good news is, studies show that women who continue to exercise through pregnancy usually reach their prepregnancy proportions sooner after delivery than their sedentary counterparts.

Women who exercise consistently during pregnancy can resume exercise postpartum as early as two weeks after delivery, assuming that they experienced a normal vaginal delivery with no complications. Exercising postpartum women have shown to have a more rapid recovery both physically and emotionally than women who do not exercise postpartum. The incidence of postpartum depression is also low.

In addition to exercise, eating nutritiously is an important part of the equation in assuring a healthy pregnancy. Pregnant women need to eat adequately and regularly to assure that the baby is getting enough glucose to sustain growth.

Symptoms of Overtraining

For the average woman, there is no reason to perform strenuous exercise during pregnancy. Pregnancy is a time to exercise moderately with goals of improving muscle tone, especially in areas affected by pregnancy, increasing flexibility to reduce the incidence of lower back problems and other pregnancy-related discomforts, and maintaining healthful fitness levels.

There are some pregnant athletes who need to maintain a higher level of fitness to continue their sport after delivery. If these women choose to exercise more rigorously during pregnancy, frequent monitoring of the baby's growth is essential and is the major determining factor for prescribing fitness throughout the pregnancy.

However, sometimes women have exercise goals that are not in keeping with a healthy pregnancy. Frequently, women who are used to exercising strenuously before pregnancy insist on continuing their strenuous regimens during pregnancy despite recommended safety guidelines. Rather than using a rating of perceived exertion to monitor their exercise intensity, they use their *preferred* exertion level instead. In other words, they are listening to their heads or egos rather than listening to their bodies. In these cases, symptoms of overtraining may surface.

Symptoms characteristic of overtraining for women include fatigue, pain, loss of motivation, increased susceptibility of injury, and common infections. When mom overtrains, her baby is also affected. If the exercise is interfering with the baby's ability to get enough nutrients or oxygen, the baby will experience slow growth. The long-term effects of slow growth are not well understood, but researchers and obstetrical health care providers believe slow fetal growth to be associated with emotional and learning disabilities in childhood.

During a rigorous exercise session, the baby may not move as much as usual. Generally, after an exercise session, the baby will move two to three times within the first 30 minutes after exercise. If a woman notices a decrease in movement after exercise, it's a good idea to have the baby medically evaluated. Once it is determined that the baby is okay, exercise intensity should be modified to be less intense and perhaps performed less often. The goals of exercise should never interfere with the goals of a healthy pregnancy.

Exercise Safety

Before starting or continuing any exercise program during pregnancy, consult your obstetrical health care provider to be sure you do not have any limitations on activity. Ask about sports or exercises that you like to do. You will want to avoid competitive sports throughout your pregnancy, however.

On the whole, any activity you like to do other than horseback riding, sky diving, or scuba diving can be continued throughout pregnancy, provided you follow certain safety guidelines, monitor exercise intensity, and adjust your level according to how you feel. Exercise to feel good, not to lose weight. Regular exercise is preferable to intermittent activity.

Dress for the weather. If it is hot outside, exercise in the morning or evening, not around noon. Layer clothing so you can decrease body temperature when heated. If it is cold outside, wear warm clothing. In general, try to avoid exercising in extreme temperatures. On very hot or cold days, exercise indoors. Also, never exercise if you have a fever. High internal body temperatures, especially in early pregnancy, are associated with birth defects. Stay out of hot tubs, too.

Be sure to eat a light, low-fat snack at least 1 hour before exercise to avoid having low blood sugar. If you typically exercise in the morning before breakfast, drink at least 8 ounces of juice before you exercise. Drink plenty of noncaffeinated fluids before, during, and after a workout. Be sure to replace fluids even if you choose swimming as an exercise activity. When you exercise in water, you can also become dehydrated.

Warning Signs

If you experience the following symptoms, stop exercising and consult your obstetrical health care provider.

Dizziness or faintness
Shortness of breath
Irregular or rapid heart beat (palpitations)
Chest pain
Difficulty walking
Decreased fetal movement
Vaginal bleeding
Uterine contractions
Leaking of vaginal fluid
Calf pain or swelling

When you exercise, wear supportive shoes and a supportive bra. The best breast support lifts your breasts inward and upward (cross your heart). Some women may find comfort in wearing two bras while exercising.

Warm up for 5 minutes by performing the activity at a slower pace. For example, if walking is your exercise, walk slowly; if cycling is your exercise, bike slowly. When exercising, avoid motions that are bouncy, jerky or high impact. Jumping and jarring motions, as well as changing directions quickly, can increase the risk of joint injury. The hormone relaxin, secreted in pregnancy, puts the pregnant woman at a higher risk for joint injury. When performing resistance exercises, never hold your breath. Be sure to exhale on the effort.

Avoid performing any exercises on your back after the first trimester. This can decrease blood flow to the baby. Avoid motionless standing for a long time. This can also decrease blood flow to the baby as well as precipitate premature labor. Exercise at an intensity at which you can talk. If you are feeling out-of-breath, chances are that your baby is not getting enough oxygen as well. Modify exercise when necessary, especially in the last trimester when the baby is growing faster and you are getting bigger. Never exercise to the point of fatigue.

Monitor heart rate during peak levels of aerobic activity to ensure that exercise intensity is within the desired range. Pregnant women should exercise at 50 to 80 percent of maximal heart rate. To calculate maximal heart rate, subtract your age from 220 then multiply by 50 percent and 80 percent to find your desired range.

Rise slowly from a sitting or lying position to prevent feeling faint or dizzy. Then slowly walk around to reestablish circulation. Always cool down for 5 to 10 minutes after exercise by slowly decreasing your pace and performing gentle stretches.

Listen to your body! Every day, you are changing. What you did yesterday might not be feasible today. Rest when you get tired. Never exercise to the point of exhaustion. Remember, if you are feeling tired and worn out, your baby is probably not getting enough glucose or oxygen.

Popular Recreational Exercises and Sports

Walking is the perfect weight-bearing exercise for pregnant women. You do not need any special equipment or training. However, during pregnancy, the increased body weight puts stress on the arches of the feet. Be sure to wear shoes with a flexible sole and good arch support.

Also, as you walk, the foot tends to move forward. For this reason, there should be enough room in your shoes for your feet to move forward without touching the toe of the shoe. If you feel any discomfort in the shins when you walk, decrease the pace. You may also find that walking twice a day for 15 minutes instead of once for 30 minutes puts less stress on the legs and feet. It also is recommended to incorporate walking into your daily routine. For example, take the stairs, park your car away from the front door, walk instead of driving to a friend's house, and so on.

Swimming is the perfect non-weight-bearing exercise for pregnant women. It's the only time you will feel light on your feet. Also, the pressure of the water on the skin improves circulation and helps reduce swelling that normally occurs in pregnancy, especially in the latter months. Another great exercise in the water is water walking. Just by walking through water, you help to strengthen the muscles of the abdomen and reduce stress on the lower back.

If you were *jogging* before getting pregnant, it is safe to continue as long as you follow the safety guidelines listed earlier. If you never jogged before, do not start now! Jogging puts a lot of stress on the joints and can be too intense for many pregnant women. A better alternative for women who choose to continue is walk-jogging. By alternating walking and jogging, you will reduce the risk of injury to the joints and exercise at an intensity that is more appropriate for you and your baby.

Because of the changes in balance that result in pregnancy, *stationary cycling* is preferable to cycling on the road. Also, when leaning forward on a bike, try to flex at the hip joint, keeping the back straight rather than bending at the waist (figure 5.1). This will help to reduce stress on the low back. Pregnant women who attend spinning classes can safely continue taking classes, provided they follow the safety guidelines and listen to their bodies. If the instructor is moving at a pace that makes you feel sore or out-of-breath, decrease the pace or rest every so often.

Aerobic exercise classes intended for the nonpregnant woman are typically inappropriate for pregnant women in the second and third trimesters. The intensity is too high, and while exercisers are getting faster and possibly more shapely, pregnant women are getting slower and bigger. A class especially developed for pregnant women is much more appropriate and leaves the pregnant woman feeling better about the changes that are occurring in her body.

The pregnant woman who has been attending *step aerobics* classes can continue to participate only in the first trimester. After that, the risk of losing one's balance or injuring joints outweighs the benefits.

In the first trimester, women who are used to taking *Pilates* can safely continue. However, after the first trimester, exercises should not be performed while lying flat on the back. Also, it is not recommended to lie on

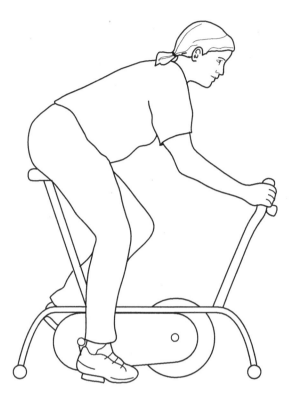

FIGURE 5.1   Flex at the hip when leaning forward on a bicycle, keeping the back straight.

the belly once the baby starts to grow and the uterus expands (about 20 weeks). Some pregnancy exercise classes incorporate Pilates exercises that require you to be on your side or on hands and knees. These exercises are safe, provided you make sure that the spine stays in the neutral position at all times.

Yoga is an excellent way to keep the body in balance during pregnancy. However, there are certain poses to avoid. Pregnant women are advised to avoid poses that require one to be inverted (upside-down). Inverting during pregnancy puts strain on the uterus and shunts blood flow away from the uterus. In the latter months of pregnancy, putting the heart below the hips also puts excess strain on the heart.

After the first trimester, a woman should avoid any poses that require being flat on her back or on her stomach (for obvious reasons). Breathing exercises are a great complement to relaxation breathing learned in preparation for labor and delivery. Stick with breathing that is slow and fluid. Avoid any breathing exercises that require you to hold your breath. Also, "breath of fire" is not recommended for pregnant women.

Women who performed *weight training* before pregnancy can continue. Pregnancy is not a good time, however, for a woman to start weight training. If you are weight training, consider reducing the weight you lift and increasing repetitions. Pregnancy is a time to maintain fitness, not strive for great gains. I recommend performing one set of each exercise for 15 to 20 repetitions. Be sure to exhale on the effort, and never hold your breath. Holding the breath while lifting weights could increase the risk of the placenta separating from the uterine wall. This could be life-threatening to both you and your baby. It is always a good idea to have a trainer work with you if you choose to continue weight training throughout your pregnancy.

The lateral motions required for *tennis* may put stress on the muscles that support the hips as well as the knees and ankles. It is best to avoid competitive sports during pregnancy, but if you are interested in playing for fun, be careful and listen to your body. Usually in the latter months of pregnancy, tennis may be too stressful on the stretching pelvis. Because of the risk of being hit in the abdomen, I do not recommend playing *racquetball* during pregnancy.

As the baby grows, the mother's center of balance changes, which could predispose her to fall while *in-line skating*. Any sport that requires balance should be avoided in the second and third trimesters of pregnancy. Remember, if you injure yourself during pregnancy, your choices of treatment are limited. So, always play it safe for the sake of you and your baby!

For *snow skiing*, the balance concerns are the same as for skating. Here, too, the risk of injury offsets the benefits of the sport. If you choose to ski despite the risks, stay on slopes that are easier than the ones you are used to. If you are used to skiing black runs, go down to blue; if you are used to skiing blue runs, go down to green. Dehydration is also a risk at higher elevations. Be sure to drink adequate amounts of water. Avoid extremes of temperature. Wear adequate clothing to stay warm, but layer clothing to avoid overheating.

Water skiing and *surfing* both carry the risk of water being forced into the vagina, which can be dangerous for a pregnant woman. These sports are not recommended at all during pregnancy.

It is against the regulations set by the Professional Association of Diving Instructors (PADI) for pregnant women to *scuba dive*. The pressure changes and increase in nitrogen may be hazardous to both mother and baby. Try *snorkeling* instead.

Walking from hole to hole while *golfing* can be tiring and dehydrating in warm weather, but other than that, golfing is fine for pregnant women. Be sure to stretch your muscles to avoid problems with the lower back.

Bowling is another sport that may put too much strain on the lower back. Use good body mechanics, stretch, and use a ball that weighs less than what you are used to. Also, never hold your breath!

If you are used to *riding horses*, continuing in the early months of pregnancy may be okay provided you do not do any jumps. However, there is always a risk of falling off of the horse, so you need to ask yourself, *Do the benefits of riding a horse outweigh the risk of injuring yourself and your baby?* There is also a concern that any activity that causes a jarring to the body in the early months of pregnancy can interfere with implantation. If you have experienced a miscarriage in the past or have infertility problems, it is probably best to avoid horseback riding altogether until after pregnancy. And of course, pregnancy is not a time to start!

The Pregnant Athlete

Women who exercise vigorously before pregnancy can continue to exercise throughout pregnancy at higher intensity levels than previously sedentary women provided they follow the exercise safety tips mentioned earlier in this chapter. It is also important to monitor the pregnancy closely to be sure that the baby is growing adequately.

While it is true that pregnant athletes can tolerate higher levels of exercise intensity, it is also important to listen to your body and modify exercise intensity when needed. The trap that many pregnant athletes fall into is pushing themselves beyond their individual tolerance levels to keep up with their prepregnancy exercise regimens.

During pregnancy, exercise goals need to change to help support the growing fetus. In the first trimester, you will probably be able to keep up with your prepregnancy regimen, but you may feel more tired and out of breath sooner than when you were not pregnant. This is your body's way of telling you to slow down. Again, listen to your body and rest when you are tired. You may find that breaking up your exercise routine into smaller time slots several times a day is easier to tolerate than trying to exercise for long periods.

In the second trimester, because of the cardiovascular changes in your body, heart rate is a poor predictor of exercise intensity, so using rating of perceived exertion is your best guide. As you increase in body weight, aerobic exercise may be more difficult to maintain.

Consider this equation: body mass × work of exercise = exercise intensity. When your body mass increases, the exercise intensity increases even when the work of the exercise session stays the same. So, during the second trimester, as your weight increases, you need to actually reduce the work of exercise to maintain the same intensity.

For many female athletes, decreasing the work of exercise is a challenge. Some women are so afraid that they will lose ground if they reduce their training intensity. However, the reverse is true. By adapting exercise regimens to meet the needs of your pregnant body, you will help reduce the risk of injury to both you and your baby.

After your baby is delivered and you return to your training schedule, you will be surprised how fast you get back. In fact, several research studies have shown that the physical changes of pregnancy seem to improve performance after delivery by strengthening the heart and lungs as well as the muscles that support the growing uterus.

Pregnancy and childbirth are similar to athletic events. Focus on modifying your training to meet the specific needs of pregnancy. If you are a runner, in the second and third trimesters of pregnancy, integrate a walk-jog regimen. As your weight increases, there is more stress on the hips, knees, and ankles. By practicing a walk-jog, you will reduce stress on these vulnerable areas of the body. Jogging in water is also a good alternative. With the increased resistance of the water, you may actually find your legs are a lot stronger after pregnancy than before.

If you are a cyclist, monitor your breathing and exercise at an intensity that allows you to continue talking. Sometimes exercising with a buddy will heighten your awareness of your ability to carry on a conversation while exercising. However, be sure that your buddy is empathetic with your pregnancy. Sometimes well-meaning friends may push you beyond your comfort level. Remind your athletic friends that you need to focus on what is good for you and your baby, not your performance schedule.

Swimming is easier to modify because rhythmic breathing will adjust naturally. But remember, *never hold your breath!* Each time you hold your breath, you are increasing intra-abdominal pressure, putting stress on the pregnancy, and decreasing oxygen to your baby.

Pregnancy is a time to maintain fitness, not make great gains. If you are a weightlifter, lower the amount of weight you are lifting and increase the number of repetitions. Lifting heavy weights can increase intra-abdominal pressure and possibly cause the placenta to separate from the uterus, which, as mentioned earlier, is a life-threatening situation for you and your baby. Also, when lifting heavy weights, blood pressure tends to increase temporarily, which is probably not a good idea in pregnancy. Be sure to hold either free weights or training bars with loose hands. Researchers find that the more tightly you hold the bars or weights, the more likely your blood pressure will elevate. Also, be sure to breathe! Holding your breath will also increase your blood pressure.

Group exercise instructors need to be aware that teaching exercise is more intense than just taking an exercise class. Take this opportunity to be a role model for modifying exercise intensity in your classes. There is nothing to be gained by pushing yourself beyond your aerobic training threshold, and you will be risking the health of both yourself and your baby.

Question: How many exercise classes can I safely teach while I am pregnant?

Answer: The nonpregnant exercise instructor is advised to limit teaching to 14 or fewer classes a week to avoid risk of injury. Of course, this depends on the type of classes being taught. During pregnancy, talk with your health care provider regarding your teaching activities. Listen to your body, modify exercise when needed, and monitor your baby for adequate growth.

Pregnancy lasts a limited time—only 9 months. Make this pregnancy about growing a healthy baby, not about trying to meet the needs of your ego. By allowing your body to adapt to the pregnancy in ways that are nurturing and healthful, you and your baby will benefit in the long run.

If you disregard your body's signals to slow down and take more time to rest, you risk injury to yourself and your baby. The consequences of injury to yourself could be such that performance after delivery is compromised. Examples include back injury, knee injury, and premature labor that requires you to be on bed rest the remainder of your pregnancy. For your baby, too much strenuous exercise could affect fetal growth and development, the effects of which may last a lifetime.

Work smarter, not harder. If you find it difficult to switch gears while you are pregnant, make a list of all the pros of exercising strenuously during pregnancy then list all of the cons. See which list is the longest and make your choice. You also may want to work with a trainer who is knowledgeable about pregnancy to prescribe a workout for you that is reasonable and safe.

Regardless of what exercises or sports you participate in or even if you have never exercised before, the following exercises should be included in your workout routine to be sure you are strengthening and stretching the muscles that are affected by pregnancy to help bring balance into your body.

Everyday Stretches

The core conditioning exercises in chapter 1 are excellent to continue throughout pregnancy. However, after the first trimester, stay away from exercises that require you to either lie flat on your back or direct you to bring your shoulders below your hips.

For best results, strengthening exercises should be done at least twice a week and may be performed every other day. Stretching exercises should be practiced as often as possible. Ideally, it is good to sequence the exercises so that you strengthen the muscle and then follow with the appropriate stretching exercise.

First, learn the common, everyday stretches. Then, start to incorporate the strengthening exercises every other day or at least twice a week. For your convenience, appropriate stretching exercises are listed after each strengthening exercise. Remember, with all exercises, listen to your body and modify exercises accordingly.

Torso Stretch

Stand in good posture and bring the arms above your head with the palms together. Cross your thumbs and pull up from under the armpit. Breathe deeply into the sides of your torso. Exhaling, lean toward the right side (figure 5.2). Inhale and return to center. Exhaling, lean toward the left side. Inhale and return to center. Repeat the exercise on both sides two more times.

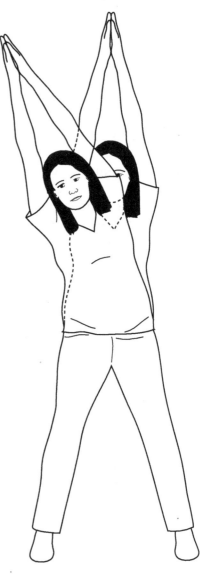

FIGURE 5.2 Torso stretch.

Shoulder Stretch

Bring your hands behind your back. Either interlace your fingers or grab the opposite wrists (figure 5.3). Breathing easily, squeeze the shoulder blades together, pulling back on the shoulders.

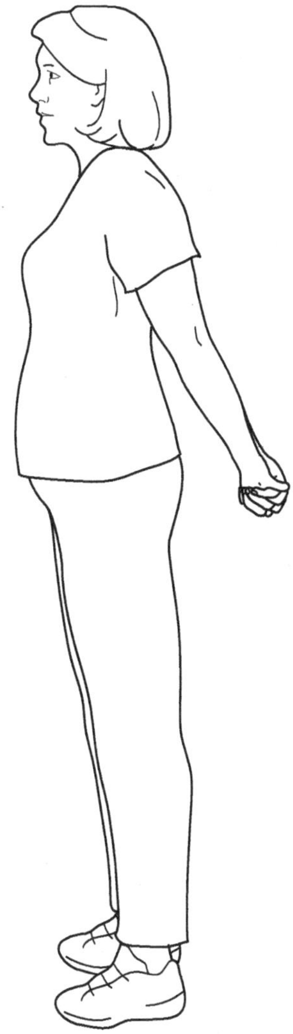

Monkey Stretch

Kneel on a mat or blanket. Bring the right leg forward with the ankle slightly in front of the knee. Place the hands on top of the right thigh and interlace your fingers (figure 5.4). Inhaling, shift your weight forward and hold the stretch while breathing normally. Hold the position for 3 to 5 breaths. Then shift your weight back toward the left knee and repeat the exercise on the same side. Perform the exercise twice on the left side.

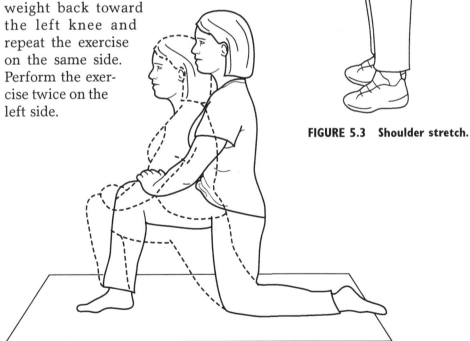

FIGURE 5.3 Shoulder stretch.

FIGURE 5.4 Monkey stretch.

Leg Extension

Sit with one leg straight and one leg bent. Flex the foot toward the head. With the hands extended alongside of the leg, lengthen the spine, keeping the inward curve of the lower back (figure 5.5). As you inhale, imagine lengthening your spine. As you exhale, release your torso toward your foot. Continue this pattern for 3 to 5 breath cycles. When you can't go any further, round the back into a forward fold for 3 to 5 breaths and slowly sit back up. Repeat the exercise with the other leg extended.

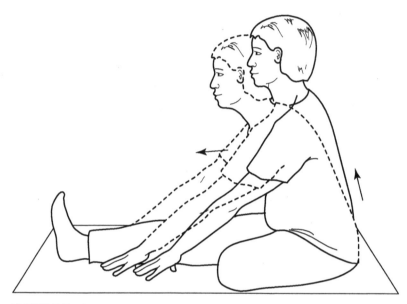

FIGURE 5.5   Leg extension.

Quadriceps Stretch

While lying on your side, bend the top knee and reach back with the hand on the same side to grab the ankle or foot (figure 5.6a). Pull the knee gently back to stretch the front of the thigh.

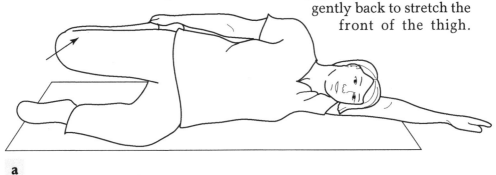

a

Hold the position for 3 to 5 breaths. Repeat the stretch on the other side.

This exercise can also be done while standing and balancing on one foot (figure 5.6b). Use the wall for balance if you need to.

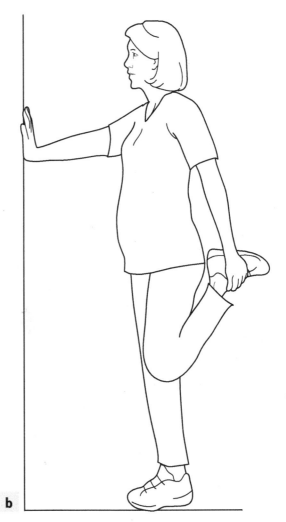

b

FIGURE 5.6 Quadriceps stretch: (a) lying on the side; (b) standing on one foot.

Squats

Separate the feet wider than hip-width apart and walk the hands toward the knees while shifting the weight to the heels of the feet (figure 5.7). Either keep the hands on the floor for balance or bring the palms together in front of the heart with the elbows pressing against the inner knees. Hold the position for 3 to 5 breaths.

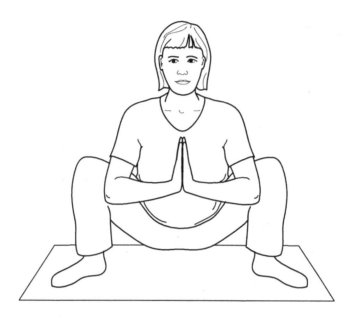

FIGURE 5.7   Squat.

Garland Pose

From a squatting position with feet hip-width apart, shift your weight to the balls of the feet. Extend the arms between the knees with the head relaxed, facing downward (figure 5.8). Hold the position for 3 to 5 breaths.

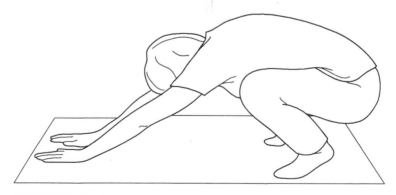

FIGURE 5.8   Garland pose.

Bound Angle

Sit with the soles of the feet together. Hold the ankles or feet with both hands. Relax the shoulders and reach the knees toward the floor (figure 5.9). Stretch up through the spine with your crown reaching toward the ceiling. Lean forward and hold the position for 3 to 5 breaths.

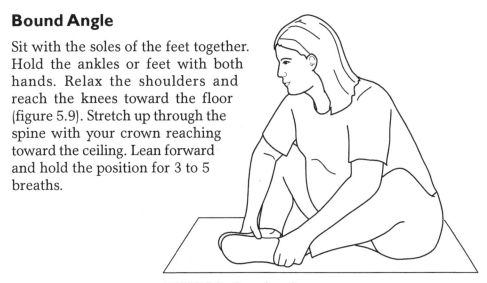

FIGURE 5.9   Bound angle.

Sitting Lateral Stretch

Sit with the right leg extended to the side and the foot flexed. The left leg is bent in front. If this is uncomfortable, keep left leg extended in front. Extend the arms to the sides at shoulder level. Inhaling, raise the left arm while the right arm reaches toward the right leg. Exhaling, lean the torso toward the right leg while reaching the left arm up and over toward the right (figure 5.10). Hold the position for 3 to 5 breaths. Repeat the stretch on the other side.

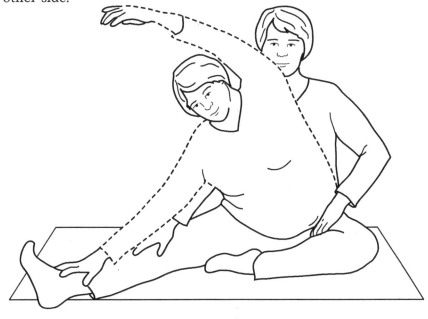

FIGURE 5.10   Sitting lateral stretch.

Neck Relaxer

Sit comfortably in a chair or on the floor. Bring both hands to the shoulders by the sides of the neck, fingers facing behind you. Inhaling, pull the shoulders forward, looking up toward the ceiling (figure 5.11). Exhale and bring head back to center.

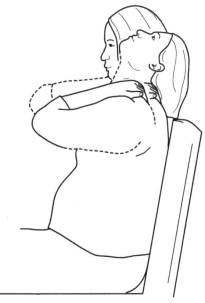

FIGURE 5.11   Neck relaxer.

Sidelying Leg Extensions

Lie comfortably on one side. Bend the top leg and bring the knee toward the shoulder. Wrap your arm around the knee, stretching the pelvic area. Release the knee and extend the leg up to the ceiling. Reach behind the leg and slowly walk your hand up the back of the leg, gently stretching the calves and hamstrings (figure 5.12). Pull up your kneecap and flex the foot for added stretch. Hold the position for 3 to 5 breaths and release. Repeat the stretch on the other side.

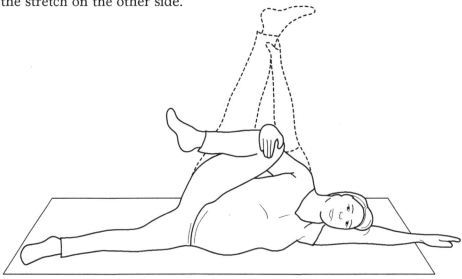

FIGURE 5.12   Sidelying leg extension.

Spine Rotation Stretch

Lie on one side with the knees bent and the top arm extended on the top hip. Reach the top arm toward the feet and then slowly rotate the arm forward, up toward the head and eventually to the opposite side at shoulder level, following with your head (figure 5.13). Keep reaching the arm, trying to get the shoulder on the floor. Hold the position for 3 to 5 breaths and then bring the arm back to the hip. Repeat the stretch on the same side, and then repeat it twice on other side.

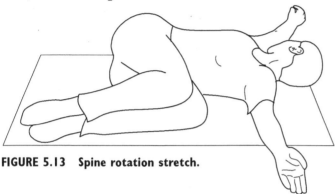

FIGURE 5.13   Spine rotation stretch.

Calf Stretch

Stand with the right leg behind you, the left knee bent to 90 degrees, and the back foot facing forward. Reach forward or place the hands on a wall (figure 5.14). Inhale and lift the right heel up. Exhale and bring the right heel down. Hold the position for 3 to 5 breaths. Repeat the stretch on the left leg.

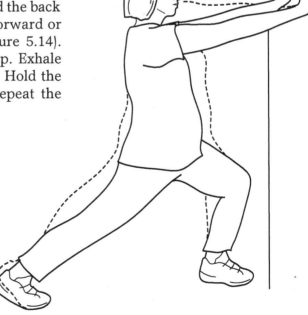

FIGURE 5.14   Calf stretch.

Sitting Hip Stretch

Sit with the soles of the feet together and the knees at a 90-degree angle. Inhale and stretch into the spine, reaching the crown of the head toward the ceiling (figure 5.15). Exhale and release forward, keeping the back straight and the head in alignment with the spine. Again, inhale to stretch up and exhale to come forward. Continue this sequence until you can't go any further and then round the back and release your head toward your feet. Hold the position for 3 to 5 breaths and slowly roll back up to good sitting posture.

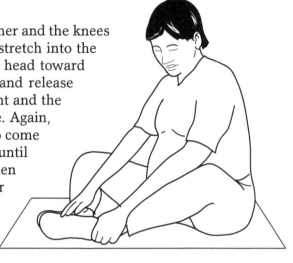

FIGURE 5.15   Sitting hip stretch.

Modified Triangle Pose

Stand with your feet comfortably spread apart, the right knee bent with feet facing toward the right, and the arms extended at shoulder level. Reach the right arm toward the right knee and lean toward the right, placing the right elbow on top of right thigh (figure 5.16). Bring the left arm up toward the left ear and stretch into the left side. Hold the position for 3 to 5 breaths. Inhale to come back to center and repeat the exercise on other side.

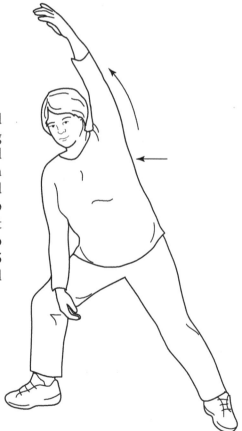

FIGURE 5.16   Modified triangle pose.

Strengthening Muscles to Support Your Baby

These exercises can be done in any order, however, it is recommended to follow the exercise with the counter stretch noted. By performing the counter stretch, you will help to keep the muscle healthy as well as prevent injury.

Belly Breathing

Sit in a comfortable position with good posture—the ears over the shoulders and the shoulders over the hips. As you inhale, relax your belly. As you exhale, pull your belly toward your spine to "hug the baby." Repeat the exercise for 20 breath cycles. Follow with a sitting hip stretch (page 90).

Cat Bows

Get into a tabletop position with your back straight and head in alignment with your torso. Keep the knees directly under your hips. As you inhale, bend your elbows and lower your chest to the floor (figure 5.17). Exhale and straighten your arms to come back up. Repeat the exercise for 10 to 12 breath cycles. Follow with shoulder and monkey stretches (page 83).

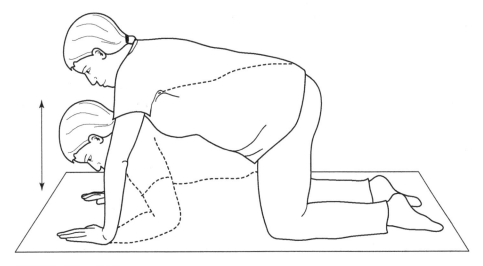

FIGURE 5.17   Cat bow.

An alternate exercise is wall push-ups. Stand about 6 inches from the wall. Place both hands on the wall at shoulder level or slightly below. As you inhale, bend your elbows and bring your chest toward the wall (figure 5.18). Exhale and straighten the arms. Repeat the exercise for 10 to 12 breath cycles.

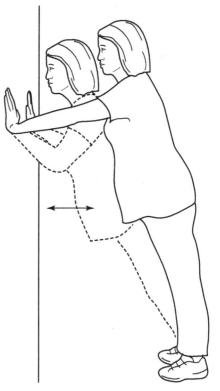

FIGURE 5.18   Wall push-ups.

Incline Plane

Sit with the legs bent and parallel to each other. Keep the feet flat on the floor. Place your hands behind your buttocks. Slide your shoulders downward, away from your ears. Exhale and lift your buttocks off the floor (figure 5.19). (Optional: Let the head extend back.) Hold the position for 3 to 5 breaths and then bring the buttocks back to floor. Repeat the exercise again. Follow with garland pose (page 86).

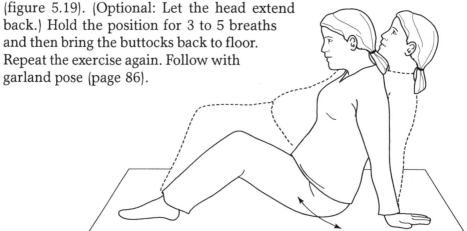

FIGURE 5.19   Incline plane.

Modified Mermaid

Sit on the right hip with the right knee facing forward and the left knee pointing up into the air with your left foot flat on the floor. Extend the right arm next to your right hip for support and your left arm on top of left knee (figure 5.20a). As you inhale, lift your right hip off the floor and bring your left arm up toward the ceiling. As you exhale, bring your left arm over to the right while looking down at right hand (figure 5.20b). Inhale and reach the left arm up again. Exhale and return to starting position. Repeat the exercise a total of 3-5 times and then switch to the other side. Follow with spine rotation stretch (page 89).

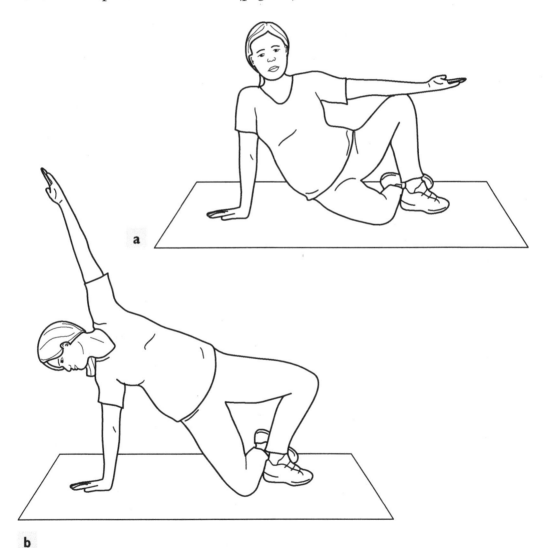

FIGURE 5.20   Modified mermaid: *(a)* **sit with the knees bent;** *(b)* **lift the hip off the floor and reach with left hand.**

Lunges

With your arms relaxed at your sides, inhale and step forward onto your right leg while bending your right knee. Keep the knee in line with your toes. Exhale and step your right leg back, bringing the legs together (figure 5.21). Repeat the exercise on the left leg. Alternate sides for a total of 10 to 12 lunges on each side. Follow with leg extension stretch (page 84).

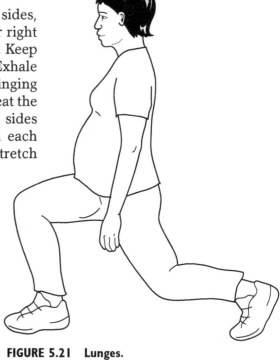

FIGURE 5.21   Lunges.

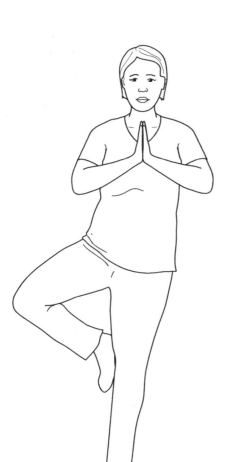

Stork Pose

Stand in good posture with the feet hip-width apart. Shift your weight onto your left leg while bringing your right foot to the left leg (figure 5.22). Keep the palms together in front of your heart center. Hold the position for as long as you can and then switch to the other leg. Follow with garland pose (page 86).

FIGURE 5.22   Stork pose.

Chair Pose

Stand with the feet hip-width apart and the arms relaxed by your sides. Bend the knees, keeping them over the heels. Reach the arms forward at shoulder level (figure 5.23). Hold the position for 3 to 5 breaths. While exhaling, squeeze the buttock muscles and return to standing position. Follow with quadriceps stretch (page 84).

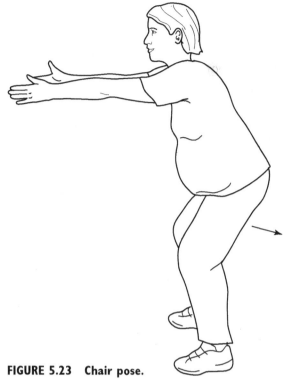

FIGURE 5.23   Chair pose.

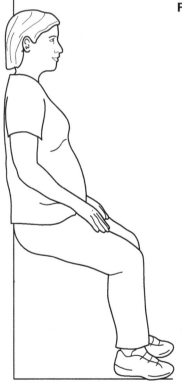

An alternate exercise is the assisted chair pose. Lean against a wall and bend the knees, sliding down the wall until the knees are at hip level (figure 5.24). Press back toward the wall and hold the position for 3 to 5 breaths.

FIGURE 5.24   Assisted chair pose.

Warrior I Pose

Bend your right knee and extend
your left leg behind you with
the left foot pointing to the side.
Extend the arms beside your ears
with the palms facing inward
(figure 5.25). Hold the position for
3 to 5 breaths. Repeat the exercise
on the other side. Follow with calf
stretch on each side (page 89).

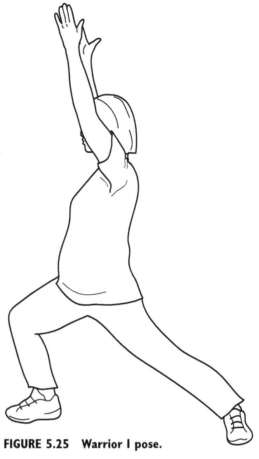

FIGURE 5.25   Warrior I pose.

Warrior II Pose

Start in a wide-legged stance with the feet parallel. Turn the right foot to
the right and bend your right knee to a 90-degree angle. Try to get the
right thigh parallel to the floor. Extend the arms out to the sides at shoulder level (figure 5.26). Look over the right arm and hold the position for
3 to 5 breaths. Repeat the exercise on other side. Follow with quadriceps
stretch (page 85).

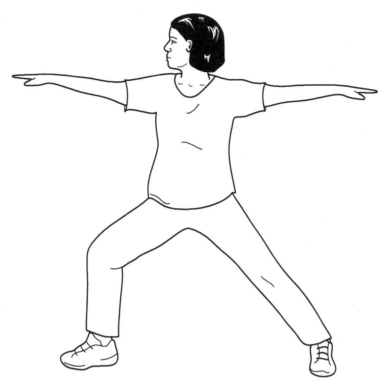

FIGURE 5.26   Warrior II pose.

Sidelying Inner Thigh Lift

Lie on your right side. Bend your left knee to the ceiling with the foot flat on the floor. Extend the right leg. As you exhale, lift your right leg and hold it in the air for 3 to 5 breaths as you breathe normally (figure 5.27). Repeat the exercise on the other side. Follow with the spine rotation stretch (page 89).

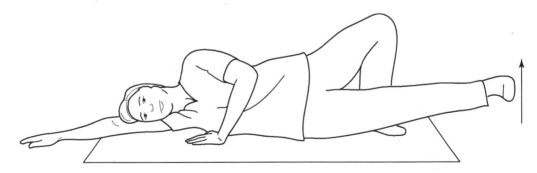

FIGURE 5.27   Sidelying inner thigh lift.

Sunbird Pose

Get into a tabletop position, with the shoulders over the wrists and the hips over the knees. If your wrists are sore, make a fist and rest on the back of the hands. Shift your weight onto one knee and extend the opposite leg (figure 5.28). Keep the back foot either on the floor or lifted no higher than the buttocks. Hold the position for 3 to 5 breaths. Repeat the exercise on the other side. Follow with garland pose (page 86).

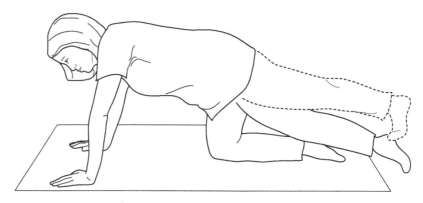

FIGURE 5.28   Sunbird pose.

Balancing Sunbird

From a tabletop position, shift your weight onto your right knee, extend your left leg behind you, and bring your right arm next to your right ear (figure 5.29). Hold the position for 3 to 5 breaths. Repeat the exercise on the other side. Follow with garland pose (page 86) and shoulder stretch (page 83).

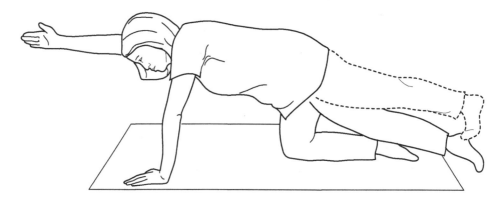

FIGURE 5.29   Balancing sunbird.

Sit-Backs

Sit with the knees apart and feet flat on the floor. Place the hands on the shins below the knees. Exhale and pull your belly toward your spine. Bring the hips forward and round the back (figure 5.30). Inhale and straighten the spine. Repeat 10 to 12 times. Follow with monkey stretch (page 83).

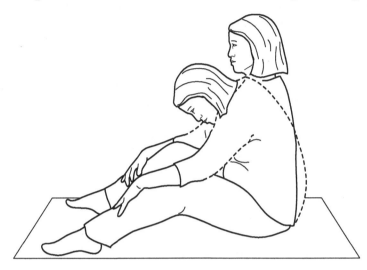

FIGURE 5.30   Sit-back.

Sit-Backs With Spinal Twist

Sit in the same position as for sit-backs. Exhale and pull the belly toward the spine, rounding the back while turning the torso to one side (figure 5.31). Inhale and straighten your spine, bringing your torso to the center. Repeat the exercise to the other side. Alternate sides for 10 to 12 times. Follow with a side-lying quadriceps stretch (page 85).

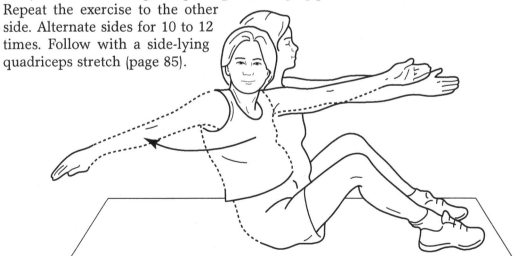

FIGURE 5.31   Sit-back with spinal twist.

Workout Schedule

The sample workout schedule shown in table 5.1 refers to timing your aerobic exercise rather than trying to accomplish a certain distance. As your pregnancy progresses, your ability to move quickly will diminish. As long as you move for a certain period of time, regardless of the intensity, you will reap the many benefits of exercise during pregnancy. For more specific instructions on exercising during each trimester of pregnancy, refer to chapters 7 through 9.

TABLE 5.1   Sample Weekly Workout Routine

Day 1	20 to 30 minutes walking, swimming, or stationary cycling Everyday stretches (can be done throughout the day)
Day 2	Two 10- to 15-minute walks Five strengthening exercises and their corresponding stretches
Day 3	20 to 30 minutes walking, swimming, or stationary cycling Everyday stretches (can be done throughout the day)
Day 4	Two 10- to 15-minute walks Five strengthening exercises (preferably different ones from the exercises done on day 2) and their corresponding stretches
Day 5	20 to 30 minutes walking, swimming, or stationary cycling Everyday stretches (can be done throughout the day)
Day 6	Two 10- to 15-minute walks Five strengthening exercises (preferably different ones from the exercises done on day 4) and their corresponding stretches
Day 7	Rest

When you ask most people why they do not exercise on a regular basis, the most frequent response is, "not enough time." Finding time to exercise is easier when you consciously make the time.

First of all, get a calendar if you do not already have one. It is a good idea to purchase a new calendar at the beginning of your pregnancy to help you manage your time as well as keep a diary of your pregnancy. This makes a great keepsake that you will want to share with your child in years to come. It also helps identify any areas of concern that might affect future pregnancies.

Fill in any scheduled activities you have planned already. Then choose a time every day that you will devote to exercise. You may want to plan one hour at a time or break it up into smaller segments. Take into account any exercise classes you are taking, times you need to walk the dog, or activities that you like to do such as dancing, biking, or swimming. Write down the times you plan to exercise for the next week. Aim to exercise aerobically (walk, swim, bike) at least 30 minutes a day as well as practice torso strengthening exercises and everyday stretches.

Daily exercise does not have to fit into one-hour blocks of time. In fact, your body is designed to perform activity throughout the day at moderate levels. It is quite healthy to exercise in 10- or 15-minute segments. Try to get at least 20 minutes of aerobic exercise a day and include exercises that strengthen and stretch muscles affected by pregnancy. The main goal is to plan for exercise to happen.

Remember, when you do not have a plan, you become a part of someone else's. Once you put yourself on the calendar, you can make additional plans around yourself. So, if your spouse or boss wants you to do something for them, just say, "I'll need to check my calendar!" They don't need to know what is already there.

Another way to find time to exercise is to recognize "exercisable moments." Let's say you are waiting for an exam in the doctor's office. That is a great time to practice belly breathing and Kegels. Other times might be standing in line at the grocery store, sitting in traffic, or riding in a bus or train.

On sunny days, park your car a little further from your destination. Walk up and down stairs instead of taking the elevator. After dinner put on music and dance with your partner. At work, use a portable phone and walk around your office while on the phone. Take a walk on your break, or walk at lunch and eat at your desk. You can also do many of the strengthening and stretching exercises included in this chapter at your desk during short breaks throughout the day. Make a walking date with a friend or ride your bike to work (first trimester only).

These are all ideas for incorporating exercise into your life. Just as you wouldn't think of going through the day without brushing your teeth, get into the habit of exercising every day. Remember to rest when you are tired. It is during rest that your body is able to enjoy all the benefits of exercise.

Meditating for Relaxation and Focus

The benefits of meditation are well documented. Regular meditation practice can reduce blood pressure, prevent and treat heart disease, reduce migraines, and decrease many stress-related symptoms. Meditation has been proven to be helpful in reducing obsessive thinking, anxiety, depression, and hostility.

During pregnancy, meditation will help you decrease stress. In labor, it will help you deal more effectively with your contractions. After delivery, meditation will assist you in dealing with the challenges of being a new mom. Meditation can be learned within a few minutes. However, the benefits of meditation come over time with practice.

Question: How does meditating prepare me for labor and delivery?

Answer: When you are in labor, your body is in control. For many women, the idea of surrendering to the body is uncomfortable. If you get nervous and stressed out during labor, you might make the uterine contractions more intense or even contribute to a longer labor. Meditation teaches you to calm down and release the need to control. When you are meditating, you are focusing your mind to relax your body so it can do what it needs to do to birth your baby. In this way, practicing meditation on a daily basis prepares you for a positive labor and delivery experience.

Getting Started

Choose a comfortable sitting position. Sit with your back straight and chin tucked in slightly to lengthen the neck. Allow the small of your back to arch slightly. Sit against a wall for support if necessary. Position the shoulders over the hips and the ears over the shoulders. Pull the abdomen inward as if to hug your baby. Breathe into the sides and back of your torso in addition to your chest. Rock briefly from side to side and front to back to establish a point at which your upper torso feels balanced on your hips. Close your eyes and breathe through your nose. If you are congested, breathe in and out through your mouth. Just make sure you are breathing!

Take a few moments to notice where your body touches the floor or chair. Notice your breath. Is it deep or shallow? Fast or slow? Use slow, three-dimensional breathing. Your chest, the sides of your rib cage, and your back should expand when you inhale and contract while you exhale.

Maintaining a passive attitude is important in promoting relaxation. Remember, as a beginner, you will have very few moments of clear concentration. Without thoughts, you would not be able to develop the ability to let them go. A passive attitude includes a lack of concern for whether you are doing it right or accomplishing goals or whether meditation is right for you. Adopt the attitude that you will sit quietly for a specified time and whatever happens is exactly what should happen.

It is not necessary to feel as though you are relaxing while you meditate to become relaxed. You may feel as though you are thinking a thousand different thoughts and are very restless. However, when you end the meditation, you will feel more relaxed.

As your mind quiets, sometimes negative emotions surface from your subconscious. If this happens, experience the feeling and then tell yourself to let it go. If you feel the need, talk with a friend or counselor about your feelings.

Finding the time and motivation to meditate is a challenge. Try to get into a habit of meditating the same time each day that you practice. Many women find it helpful to meditate before going to bed. This may help you to sleep more restfully.

Meditation Poem

Recite this poem to yourself several times and notice how it makes you feel.

May the long-time sun shine upon you,
All love surround you,
And the pure light within you
Guide your way on.

—*Old Indian Chant*

Meditation Exercises

In general, any amount of time spent meditating is more relaxing than not meditating at all. Start out with 5 minutes a day. Gradually, you may want to increase the amount of time to 20 or 30 minutes once or twice a day.

Breath Counting Meditation

Sit in good posture and take several deep breaths. Either close your eyes or look at a spot on the floor. Your eyes may or may not be focused. Inhale and count to 4, pause for 1 count, then exhale for 4 counts. After you exhale, pause for 1 count and repeat the cycle.

If you would like to, expand your inhalation and exhalation to 6 counts and then to 8 counts. Be sure that you inhale and exhale evenly. If your mind slips into other thoughts, acknowledge the thoughts and then come back to counting the breath.

Mantra Meditation

Select a word or syllable that you like. It may mean something to you or just be a nonsense syllable that has a pleasant sound. Sit in good posture and take some deep breaths. Say the word or syllable silently to yourself over and over within your mind. When your thoughts stray, come back to your mantra. Let your mantra make its own rhythm as you say it over and over again. Try saying the mantra aloud and notice how you feel. Is it more relaxing to say it silently or out loud?

Remember, practice meditation with awareness. If you find that repeating the mantra becomes mechanical, notice how your body feels and then come back to the mantra. You can also change your mantra if you find your mind wandering off.

Om Meditation

The sound of the earth spinning is said to be "om." Researchers have found that people who recite this during meditation experience a natural lowering of the blood pressure. This type of chanting also helps to reduce the risk for sinus congestion and infection.

This is a four-part meditation: AH–OH–MMM–pause. Take a deep breath and sound out all four parts. Continue for at least 10 cycles and then sit quietly and notice how you feel.

At first, you may feel silly making these sounds. However over time you will feel the vibrations resonate throughout your body and leave you feeling open and relaxed. Try reciting this meditation at different octaves and notice how they affect different parts of your body.

Gazing

Find an object that you like to look at: a candle, stone, piece of wood, or anything else you feel is appropriate. Sit in good posture and take a few deep breaths. Set your object at eye level. Look at it carefully. Keep your eyes soft and relaxed. Allow yourself to become totally involved with the exploration of your object as though you had never seen it before. If thoughts or words you associate with the object pop up, simply notice them and let them go. Return your attention to the object. If you like this meditation, take your object with you when you are in labor to keep you focused during contractions.

Humming Meditation

According to Swedish scientists, humming is an effective way of increasing ventilation to the sinuses. This is important news for pregnant women, because pregnancy frequently causes swelling of the mucous membranes that line the sinuses, increasing the risk of sinus infections.

Sit in a comfortable position with good postural alignment, keeping the shoulders over the hips and the ears over the shoulders. Breathe in and out through the nose. If this is not possible, then breathe through the mouth. During exhalation, make a humming sound and sustain it until the end of the exhalation phase of your breath. While inhaling, just relax and take in as much air as possible. Try humming at a variety of octaves and notice whether you feel any differences in the sinuses.

Continue this exercise for at least 10 cycles. Sit quietly and notice how you feel. If you also want to strengthen your abdominal muscles, during exhalation pull your belly button toward your spine and during inhalation relax your belly. Kegels also can be integrated, tightening the muscles around the birth canal during exhalation and relaxing during inhalation.

Rainbow Meditation

Your body has seven major energy centers, called *chakras* (figure 6.1). These centers correspond with different energy frequencies in the body. Chakras are likened to whirlpools of energy and are assigned different colors of the rainbow.

Sit in a comfortable position. First try to visualize your energy centers as little suns radiating light energy from the centers outward. Start with the root chakra and work your way up to the seventh or crown chakra. Then see if you can visualize the colors of each energy center.

Take your time and move your focus at your own pace. Notice whether one center shines brighter than another. If you find that one center shines less than the others, spend some time just focusing your energy toward that chakra. You can also imagine pulling energy from the earth, up your spine, and then into the chakra that needs more attention.

Once you have completed this meditation, sit quietly and notice how you feel. If something does not feel right, go back and visualize that area of your body again.

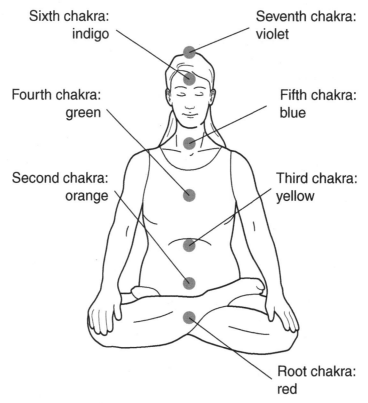

Sixth chakra: indigo

Seventh chakra: violet

Fourth chakra: green

Fifth chakra: blue

Second chakra: orange

Third chakra: yellow

Root chakra: red

FIGURE 6.1   The seven major chakras of the body.

Preparing for Labor Meditation

Record this meditation on a cassette tape or CD, then practice it while listening to the sound of your voice.

Sit comfortably in a chair or lie on your left side with a pillow under your head and a pillow between your knees. Gently close your eyes and notice your breath. Slowly breathe in and out through your nose. If it is difficult to breathe through your nose, breathe through your mouth.

As you inhale, feel your belly expand. As you exhale, feel your belly relax. Breathe slowly and easily, expanding your belly as you inhale and relaxing your belly as you exhale. Follow the rhythm of your breath.

Now, inhale slowly to the count of four—1-2-3-4. Pause. As you exhale, count backward—4-3-2-1. Pause. Keep counting as you inhale and then as you exhale, pausing briefly at the end of each inhale and then the end of each exhale, cycling the breath.

Now, inhale to the count of five—1-2-3-4-5. Pause. As you exhale, count backward—5-4-3-2-1. Pause. Continue breathing slowly and deeply. As you breathe, stay focused . . . stay relaxed . . . stay with your breath.

Continue counting your breath, breathing smoothly and easily. Breathe softly and fully, feeling the movement of your belly massaging your internal organs. With each breath, let your body, breath, and mind become one.

Bring awareness to your face. Notice any tension in your forehead. Try to make your forehead smooth and relaxed. Breathe relaxation into the space between your eyebrows. Feel your cheeks relaxing, and let go of any tension. Your jaw will begin to relax. Feel your jaw release until your lips begin to open slightly.

Take another deep breath and feel the relaxation spread into your neck, shoulders, and down your arms. As you exhale, imagine tension leaving with the breath. Your neck is loose and relaxed.

Relax your shoulders. Feel your shoulders soften and drift away from your ears as you feel more and more relaxed. Breathe relaxation into your arms, hands, and fingers. Allow the fingers to unfold, relaxing deeper and deeper with each breath. Feel the warmth of blood flowing down your arms, into your hands, and through your fingertips.

As you exhale, feel the relaxation spread to your chest, abdomen, and buttocks. Release tension as you continue to breathe slowly and deeply. Surrender to the breath. After inhaling, exhale and release.

Breathe relaxation down your legs. Let go of tension in the backs of your thighs, your knees, and your calves. Relax your feet. Wiggle your toes and then relax. Take a breath and notice the feeling of warmth flowing down your legs, into your feet, and through your toes.

With each breath, imagine breathing in peace and calm while exhaling fear and tension. Be like ice melting in the sun . . . hold onto nothing.

Hold onto nothing but your breath. Notice the breath as it flows through your body. Imagine breathing relaxation into your abdomen and spreading it through your arms and legs. Be like a water lily swaying in the current of a stream. Imagine yourself swaying in one direction as you inhale and then the other as you exhale. Move gracefully with the breath, inhaling peace, inhaling calm, inhaling total relaxation.

Now, be in this moment. Be with your breath. Feel the miracle of life growing inside of your body. Breathe deeply and slowly. Continue to follow each breath . . . become one with your breath . . . become one with your baby.

Feel the special connection you have with your baby. As you inhale, imagine oxygen flowing through your bloodstream, then through the umbilical cord to the baby inside of you. As you exhale, imagine any impurities leaving with the breath. Inhale health for both you and your baby.

Imagine what it feels like to float inside a warm, protective womb, listening to your mother's heart beat, the sound of water gently moving around you. Feel your arms and legs floating in the amniotic fluid as your mother gently rocks you with every movement of her body. Feel loved, feel safe, feel contented . . . be in this moment.

Carrying a new life inside of you connects you to every pregnant woman past, present. and future. Take a few moments to embrace this amazing experience with your heart, creating the next generation as well as generations to come. Embrace the miracle that you are, that your baby is, and honor your body. Say to yourself, *My body is feeling healthy and strong. Each time I relax, my body becomes stronger. My body is strong and capable. When the time is right, I trust that my body will safely birth my baby.*

Take a breath and imagine yourself going into labor. You feel excited, confident, and relaxed. As your uterus prepares for the delivery of your baby, breathe deeply and calmly.

Imagine each contraction of the uterus like a wave, gradually building to a peak and then slowly subsiding. Take a breath at the beginning of each contraction and continue to breathe slowly and rhythmically as you let go of fear and let go of tension. Stay with the breath until the contraction subsides and continue to breathe in relaxation and breathe out tension. Let the breath nourish and relax you. Go with the flow of your breath, go with the flow of your body. Be in the moment and then let it go.

Now, imagine holding your beautiful baby in your arms. Look deeply into your baby's eyes. Feel the special bond between you and your baby . . . know that your baby feels it too. Give your baby a kiss and imagine your baby smiling, happy and contented. Feel the happiness, feel the contentment, and feel yourself smiling too. Cherish the moment.

Take a deep breath and start to slowly come back to your body. Stay with your breath, slow and easy, as you slowly drift back into the here and now, back into this room. With each breath, you feel refreshed and renewed. Gradually become aware of your surroundings. Stay peaceful and calm.

The next time you feel tense or discomfort in your body, try to focus your mind on the breath. Breathe deeply, inhaling relaxation and exhaling tension. Remember, the power to create calm in your body resides within you.

Begin to slowly move your body. Stay with your feelings of peace and calm as you become more awake, more aware, feeling prepared to deal with the challenges of the day. When you are ready to get up, walk around slowly to reestablish your equilibrium.

chapter 7

Adjusting Actively to the First Trimester

Morning sickness is really a misnomer. Many women in the early months of pregnancy get all-day sickness or occasional sickness. Regardless of when you get sick, nausea or vomiting during pregnancy can put a damper on your best intentions to exercise.

The most common theory of why nausea and vomiting during pregnancy occurs is the rise in the hormone human chorionic gonadotropin (HCG) or Beta-HCG and other hormones. Pregnancy hormones also increase the sense of smell, making expectant moms more sensitive to odors. This sensitivity can lead to nausea as well as an upset stomach. Stress also seems to exacerbate symptoms.

It's hard to say why some women have more nausea and vomiting than others, but those who tend to experience morning sickness include women carrying multiple births, who have a history of motion sickness, who get migraines, and those with a history of nausea and vomiting on birth control pills.

Vitamin and mineral deficiencies, specifically vitamin B_6 and calcium, are also suspect for causing nausea and vomiting during pregnancy. Researchers are also looking at toxins in certain foods. It is not unusual for pregnant women to be averse to certain foods, especially meats that carry many parasites and pathogens.

Fatigue increases during the early months of pregnancy because of hormonal influences. For some women, this is the first sign of pregnancy, and it is important to honor your body and rest when you are tired. However, if you can find a convenient time to exercise when you are not tired, you may discover that mild to moderate exercise actually gives you more energy in the long run. Exercise also helps you sleep more soundly.

Tips for the First Trimester

If you tend to get nauseated in the morning, wait until evening after you exercise to take your prenatal vitamins. Eat a few crackers before you get out of bed, and eat small, frequent meals throughout the day. Sea bands, commonly found at drug stores, may help to reduce nausea by pressing on acupressure points on the wrist. There is also some evidence that ginger helps stave off nausea. Try different strategies and see what works for you. The good news is that nausea in pregnancy usually disappears by the eighteenth week of pregnancy.

Be sure to drink nonacidic juice such as apple juice in the morning before you exercise to prevent hypoglycemia which may make you feel tired, light-headed, and nauseated.

Avoid exercises that require you to lie flat on your back if you ate within two hours of exercise. Do you remember your mother warning you not to swim after a meal? When you exercise, blood flow is pulled away from your internal organs to the working muscles. If you have just eaten a meal and you exercise, digestion will slow and your stomach may feel upset. Taking a walk after eating will help the digestive process because gravity helps push food downward in the digestive tract. Exercising on your back after you eat a meal, however, may cause the food to move backward and not only cause stomach upset but heartburn as well.

Drink lots of cold water before, during, and after exercise. Sometimes the coldness of the water will numb your stomach. Suck on ice pops or anything cold for a snack.

In the early months of pregnancy, your body needs extra rest to adjust to the changes in pregnancy. Listen to your body and rest when you are tired. Try to take a nap sometime during the day even if it means putting your head on your desk for 10 to 15 minutes.

You may feel as if you have low energy in early pregnancy as well as in the last few months. Try exercising for short periods several times throughout the day instead of exercising in a large block of time. This will help your body conserve energy and will also help to build endurance.

Your body is made to fuel and burn. Ideally, you will eat what you need for the next several hours and then after you have burned the calories you've eaten, you will replenish your body again. Eat six small meals throughout the day to keep your blood sugar up. Drink lots of water to keep your body hydrated. Low blood sugar, as well as dehydration, will tend to make you tired.

When you eat refined sugars, your body is stimulated to produce more insulin, which helps your cells metabolize the sugar for energy. Usually, the faster the blood sugar goes up, the faster it will drop. When your blood sugar falls, you feel tired. The way to counteract this cycle is to eat the more complex sugars found in fruits and high-fiber carbohydrates such as whole-wheat flour and grains. Eating protein with carbohydrates also will delay absorption of the sugars and decrease the tendency to have sharp increases and decreases in blood sugar levels. So, eat more protein and fewer refined carbohydrates. Fatigue might also result from anemia, which is common in pregnancy. Eating foods high in iron such as spinach, raisins, and liver will increase iron in your system and help to prevent anemia. Iron supplements may also be necessary. Check with your health care provider.

Eat some fat. Like protein and complex carbohydrates, fat also helps keep blood sugar levels even. Fat is also important for absorbing fat-soluble vitamins such as A, D, and E. The most healthful kind of fat to eat is found in vegetable oils such as olive oil.

Avoid caffeine. Caffeine tends to give you a temporary rush of energy, but then leaves you feeling tired when it wears off. Caffeine also causes dehydration, causing more fatigue. Read labels on bottled drinks and check for caffeine. You may be surprised to find how many products have caffeine in them. In addition to coffee and tea, think about sodas, chocolate, and iced tea.

When circulation is sluggish, you may also feel sluggish, especially during pregnancy. Exercise in water and practice yoga to help improve circulation and restore energy in the body. Avoid sitting for a long time, which also tends to slow circulation.

Sometimes we expect more from ourselves than others expect from us. If your level of anxiety is directed related to the pile of laundry in your hamper, make a weekly plan of household chores. Spread your chores out over the week instead of trying to do too much in one day. For example, do the laundry on Monday, shop for food on Tuesday, vacuum on Wednesday, and so on. Ask family members to help you when you need it. And remember, it is not the worst thing in the world if you have to turn your underwear inside out!

Fatigue and nausea are common in the first trimester. However, if you are vomiting excessively or find it difficult to perform activities of daily living, talk with your health care provider for additional suggestions as well as medications that may help you get through this passing phase. The key to anything unpleasant is to realize the impermanence of all things, including fatigue and nausea. Just keep saying to yourself, *This too will pass;* eventually it will.

Hang in there! The good news is that in the second trimester of pregnancy, you will have an increased appetite and more energy as the body adjusts to the hormones of pregnancy. Communicate with your partner about how you feel. With all the changes in early pregnancy, it is not unusual to want to refrain from sex and intimacy. Reassure your partner that usually in the second trimester the desire for intimacy and sex drive return in full force!

Exercising on a Fitness Ball

By far, the most important area of your body to strengthen and tone before, during, and after pregnancy is your torso. Without strong abdominal and back muscles, you risk injuring your back and developing poor posture throughout the rest of your pregnancy. Bad habits are hard to break!

Muscles of the sides are also important in helping to support the growing uterus and preventing additional stress on your body. Exercising on a fitness ball is a fun way to strengthen your torso without putting strain on the pelvis and knees, which become vulnerable during pregnancy.

Just by sitting on the fitness ball, you engage all of the muscles that support the growing uterus. In addition to the exercises included in this chapter, try to sit on the ball as much as you can throughout the day to strengthen your core. If you feel any back discomfort, that means your muscles are tired and need to rest. Many people use fitness balls to sit at their desk or to watch television. Be creative!

When purchasing a fitness ball, find one that fits your height and be sure to read the instructions on how to inflate and store it properly. As you sit on the fitness ball, make sure your knees are in line with your hips and your knees are over your ankles (figure 7.1). Your feet should be about hip-width apart.

The following exercises can be practiced separately or easily integrated into your exercise regimen.

Belly Breathing

Sit comfortably on the fitness ball. Inhale and allow the abdomen to expand. As you exhale, contract your abdominal muscles to force the breath out. Imagine pulling your belly button toward your spine. Try to perform 20 abdominal contractions. Rest and do 20 more.

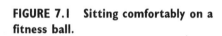

FIGURE 7.1   Sitting comfortably on a fitness ball.

For a belly breathing variation that works the quadriceps too, place the fitness ball against a sturdy wall at the level of your lower back. With your back to the ball, lengthen through the torso and lean against the ball with your knees bent and hip-width apart (figure 7.2). Perform belly breathing, pulling your belly button to your back, while keeping the ball between your back and the wall. Try to perform this exercise 20 times. Eventually try to build to 2 sets of 20 with at least 2 minutes of rest in between sets. Afterwards, perform the quadriceps stretch (page 85) to release tension on the thighs.

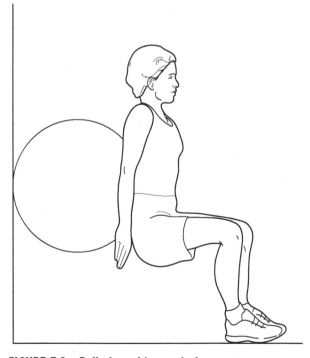

FIGURE 7.2   Belly breathing variation.

This is also a good time to practice Kegel exercises. Practicing Kegel exercises will help you strengthen and tone pelvic floor muscles, improve comfort during the later stages of pregnancy, prevent or alleviate urinary incontinence, speed up the healing process after an episiotomy, and improve sexual satisfaction.

Take a breath. While exhaling, gradually (to the count of 5) tighten the muscles around your vaginal opening as if to pull it up toward the inside of your belly button. Be sure to relax your shoulders, neck, and jaw. Only your pelvic floor muscles are tight. Inhale and relax. Perform at least 20 Kegels a day.

Question: I have exercised for years and now when I exercise, even a little bit, I get out of breath. Is that normal?

Answer: The brain regulates the oxygen–carbon dioxide balance. When you have too much carbon dioxide, the brain tells the respiratory center to breathe faster to get rid of it so more oxygen can be taken in and delivered to your baby. This gives you a feeling of being out of breath and is most common during aerobic type exercises such as walking and biking, but can happen during any exercise session. The hormones in pregnancy lower the carbon dioxide threshold in the brain, so as soon as a moderate amount builds up, you need to take quick, shallow breaths. Listen to your body. If you are feeling out of breath, chances are your baby is not getting a good supply of oxygen. When you exercise, you should be able to talk, but you shouldn't be able to sing!

Hip Circles

While sitting on the fitness ball, move the hips slowly forward and backward and then side to side. Circle the hips in one direction twice and then in the other direction twice.

Torso Turns

This exercise concentrates on working the oblique muscles of the torso. Sit on the ball with arms out to your sides at shoulder level and your wrists slightly lower than the shoulders. Exhale and turn to the right (figure 7.3). Inhale and return to center. Exhale and turn to the left. Inhale and return to center. Repeat the exercise 16 times total (8 to each side). Rest and, if you want to, perform another set.

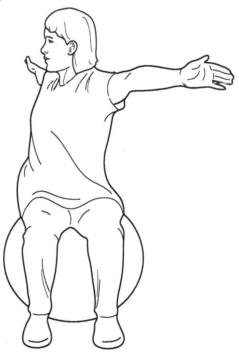

FIGURE 7.3 Torso turn.

Single-Leg Balance

Sit on the exercise ball in good posture. Extend the right leg in front with the heel resting on the floor and the arms extended out to the sides at shoulder level. Lift the right foot off the floor (figure 7.4) and hold the position for 3 to 5 breaths. Relax and repeat the exercise on the other side.

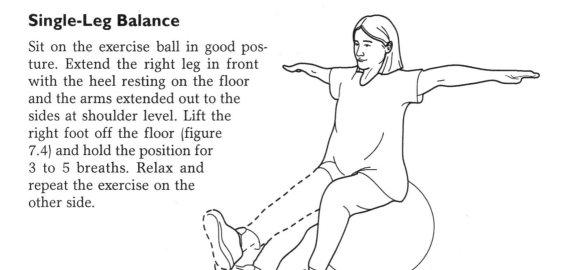

FIGURE 7.4   Single-leg balance.

Single-Leg Balance With Torso Rotation

Start in the same position as in single-leg balance. The right foot can be either on the floor or lifted slightly above the floor. As you exhale, rotate the torso to the right and stay in this position for 3 to 5 breaths (figure 7.5). As you inhale, return to center and relax. Repeat the exercise to the other side.

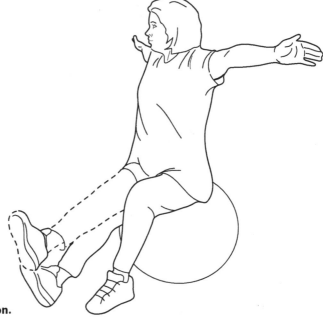

FIGURE 7.5   Single-leg balance with torso rotation.

Question: When I exercise, I feel a pull on the sides of my abdomen. Should I be concerned?

Answer: Your uterus is suspended by two ligaments. As the uterus starts to grow at the end of the first trimester, there is a pulling sensation usually in one side or the other. The pulling sensation may be intensified when you rotate your torso during exercise. If you feel this, lean into the side where you are experiencing discomfort and take some deep breaths. For more relief, put ice over the area. After about the middle of your second trimester, this sensation usually goes away.

Walk-Outs

This exercise is for women in the first trimester and postpartum women only.

Sit on the exercise ball and either hold the ball with both hands or cross your hands across your chest. As you inhale, pull your abdomen toward your spine and slowly walk your feet forward until your lower back is resting on the ball (figure 7.6). Keep the abdominal muscles tight and walk your feet in toward the ball to sit back up. Repeat the exercise for a total of 12 sets.

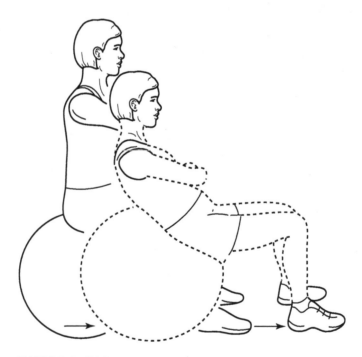

FIGURE 7.6 Walk-out.

Abdominal Crunches on the Ball

This exercise is for women in the first trimester and postpartum women only.

Perform a walk-out and keep your lower back pressed into the ball. Lightly interlace your fingers behind your head. Keep your head in good alignment as it rests in your hands. As you exhale, pull the abdomen toward the spine and lift your head and shoulders (figure 7.7). Keep the elbows out to the sides and the chin about two inches from your chest so the head is kept in proper alignment. Inhale and release back to the starting position. Do about 15 to 20 crunches. Rest and repeat again.

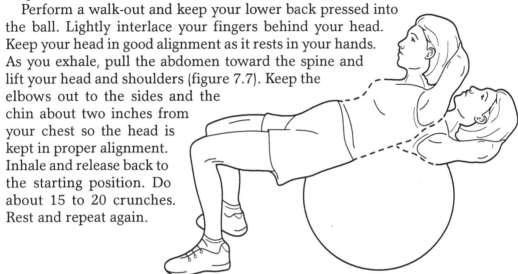

FIGURE 7.7   Abdominal crunch on the ball.

Oblique Crunches

This exercise is for women in the first trimester and postpartum women only.

Start in the same position as for abdominal crunches. As you exhale, bring the right shoulder toward the left knee (figure 7.8). Inhale and return to the starting position. Exhale and perform an oblique crunch with the left shoulder reaching toward the right knee. Alternate right and left sides for a total of 15 to 20 times on each side. Rest and repeat one more set of 15 to 20 repetitions.

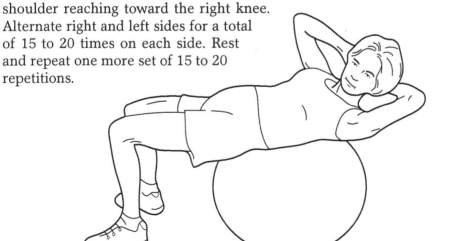

FIGURE 7.8   Oblique crunch.

Balancing on the Ball

Sit on the ball with good posture next to a chair or table. Hold onto the chair or table with one hand as you lift both feet off the floor. Try to balance while you take your hand away from the chair or table (figure 7.9). Hold the position for 3 to 5 breaths and relax. Try again. Hold the arms out to the sides while balancing or hold the arms in front of you. Find a position for your arms that helps you balance.

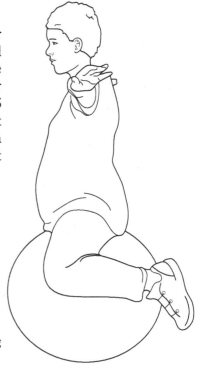

FIGURE 7.9   Balancing on the ball.

Side Stretches on the Ball

Kneel on a mat on the right side of the ball. With your left arm, reach over the ball to the floor on the other side. Extend your right leg and try to balance (figure 7.10). Stretch into your right arm, lifting it up to the ceiling and bringing it beside the right ear. Hold the position for 3 to 5 breaths and then relax. Repeat 3 more times and then switch sides.

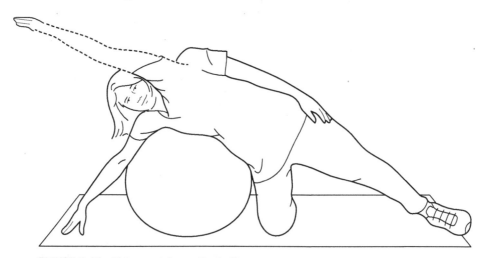

FIGURE 7.10   Side stretch on the ball.

Leg variation: If you find balancing on the ball easy, try to extend both legs while stretching the arm next to your ear (figure 7.11).

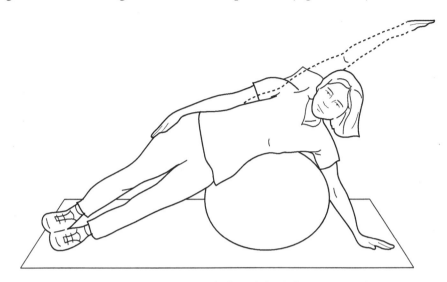

FIGURE 7.11 **Side stretches on the ball with both legs extended.**

chapter 8

Staying Motivated Through the Second Trimester

As hormones level off in the second trimester, you will begin to feel more energized. Pregnant women report feeling more like their old selves at this time. Even though you feel like doing more, exercise moderately and follow the safety guidelines, which include staying off of your back when you exercise.

This chapter will help you understand the changes that occur during the second trimester as well as reasons for exercise modifications. This is an exciting time in your pregnancy. Usually by 20 weeks of pregnancy, you start to feel your baby move. Read the suggestions for monitoring fetal movement to assess fetal well-being and learn about common symptoms of premature labor. As mentioned in the previous chapter, you will also find that your sex drive returns, so be sure to check out the section on making love during pregnancy.

In the first trimester of pregnancy, the fetus develops everything he or she needs to be a person—arms, legs, toes, ears, and so on. By the beginning of the second trimester, the fetus starts to grow larger in size. You may notice your abdomen expanding as if it just popped out overnight. You know those maternity clothes that you thought would never fit you? Guess what! Now you will actually start to fill them out. This is also a good time to begin your baby book. Save ultrasound pictures of your baby and have your partner take pictures of you to show your progression through pregnancy. Keep a pregnancy diary of thoughts, feelings, and significant events. These make great keepsakes for your child in years to come. Every day you are changing and the baby is growing, enjoy each and every moment. There is a saying in Latin, *Carpe diem*—seize the day!

Stay Off Your Back

The inferior vena cava is the principal vein that runs up the right side of your body and brings blood flow from the legs and abdominal organs to the heart and lungs, where it gets rid of the carbon dioxide. After the blood is oxygenated, it then flows through the aorta back to your body as well as to your baby.

Any pressure on the inferior vena cava interferes with blood flow getting to your heart and lungs and results in less blood going through the aorta to your baby. It also happens that when you exercise, blood is shunted from the abdominal organs, including your uterus, to the working muscles.

When you lie on your back, your growing uterus presses on the inferior vena cava, reducing the amount of blood flow to the baby. In most cases, the baby can handle the reduction in blood flow for a short while. However, when you exercise while lying flat on your back, you not only restrict blood flow, you also shunt blood away from the baby. This further reduction in blood flow might be too much for the baby to handle.

While researchers believe that fit pregnant women deliver higher oxygen saturations to their babies, it is hard to determine how much shunting of the blood is too much. So, regardless of how fit you are, it's better to err on the side of caution. You are much better off just finding alternative ways to exercise without lying flat on your back in the second and third trimesters of pregnancy.

The biggest concern for active women once they pass the first trimester is how to strengthen the abdominal muscles without lying flat on the back. Many of the exercises previously mentioned, including exercises on the fitness ball, can be done without lying flat on the back.

Question: I get light-headed when I stand up quickly from a sitting position. Is this something I should be concerned about?

Answer: The hormones in pregnancy cause your blood vessels to dilate. When you stand up quickly, the blood tends to rush to your feet and away from your head, causing you to feel light-headed. One way to avoid this is to get up slowly, taking deep breaths as you go. If dizziness continues despite getting up slowly, avoid exercises that require you to alternate sitting and standing, and report to your health-care provider.

Also, what you do every day counts! While performing any activity be conscious of what is happening in your torso. Imagine hugging your baby with your abdomen. Try to stay in good posture most of the time whether standing or sitting. When sitting on a chair, allow your back to keep you upright rather than leaning against the back of the chair.

When evaluating any exercise during pregnancy, ask yourself, *Does the benefit of the exercise outweigh the risks?* If you don't know, ask your health care provider. Why take unnecessary risks?

Question: I get pain in my wrists when I exercise on all fours in the table-top position. What can I do?

Answer: Nerve compression syndrome, or carpal tunnel, is common during pregnancy because of the postural changes in the upper body and increase in water retention in the wrists. To help alleviate symptoms, refer to chapter 2. To continue exercising, make a fist with both hands and rest the hands on the backs of the fingers between the knuckles instead of on the heels of the hands (see the illustration).

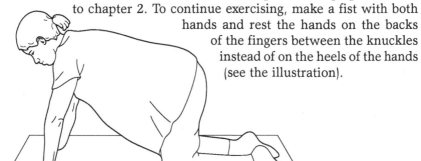

Reclaiming Your Energy

Everything in the universe is made up of energy. Heat and light are two fundamental energies needed to sustain life. Food has energy that feeds our bodies. Every thought, feeling, and action is a form of energy, and everything we come in contact with has energy that affects us in one way or another.

Sleep is a great healer. It allows our bodies to reenergize for 8 to 10 hours each night. Food also affects our energy levels. In your diet, try to eat 45 to 65 percent carbohydrates, 20 to 35 percent fat, and 10 to 35 percent protein. Try to drink 8 to 10 glasses of water a day. Small, frequent meals also help to keep your blood sugar level even.

Another energy zapper is environmental chaos. Surround yourself with beauty! Listen to sounds that are soothing. Pregnancy is a good time to get rid of clutter around the house and notice how light you feel.

Become aware of energy-draining emotions such as fear, depression, worry, and anger. Everything is thought. When you are feeling any of these emotions, try to acknowledge your feelings and then choose to let them go. Focus on your breath and practice the relaxation breathing techniques you learned in chapter 3 and the meditations described in chapter 6.

Visualize blowing up a balloon, putting your feelings into the balloon and watching it climb into the sky until it is out of sight. If you are feeling overwhelmed, you may need to seek help from a counselor or therapist. Ask your health care provider for recommendations.

Try to avoid negative people who tend to drain your energy. Instead, spend time with people who feed your soul! Notice friends and family members who tend to make you feel good about yourself. Seek out other pregnant women with whom you can identify by attending prenatal exercise and childbirth classes. Check with your local hospital or fitness center for classes in your area. Ask about instructor credentials. Instructors working with pregnant women should be certified in the areas of pre- and postnatal fitness or childbirth education.

Try to exercise at least 20 minutes every day. The sluggish circulation in pregnancy tends to make you feel tired. But once you start exercising and circulation improves, you will find you feel more energized.

Question: My legs cramp up at night. Do you have any suggestions for relief?

Answer: Leg cramps occur when circulation is affected, muscles are tense, or there is an imbalance of calcium and phosphorus. If circulation is the cause, exercises such as walking and swimming are excellent ways to improve circulation. Also see chapter 2 for tips on maintaining good posture when lying on your side. Sometimes when lying sideways with the knees together, you may cut off the circulation to the upper leg. Stretching exercises of the calves and hamstrings help reduce tension. If you drink lots of sodas, you probably have a calcium–phosphorus imbalance. Stop drinking sodas and start drinking more water.

Stick with mild to moderate exercise. There is no reason to exercise to the point of fatigue. As your weight increases from the growing fetus, you will find pregnancy to be an aerobic experience in itself, because you are overloading every day!

In addition to aerobic exercise, focus on exercises that help you become stronger and more flexible. Refer to chapter 5 for exercises to practice. Also, take at least 20 minutes every day to rest on your side and notice your baby's movements.

Counting Fetal Movements

Fetal movement is the best indicator of fetal well-being. When movement decreases, it is usually a sign that the baby is having some type of difficulty.

Fetal movements are typically felt by 18 to 20 weeks gestational age. Initially, the movements are somewhat erratic and feel like little flutterings or "butterflies" in the lower abdomen. The term used for this is *quickening*. As the baby gets bigger, the movements become stronger and more regular. After about 32 weeks, the baby has less room to move, so movements are experienced more as squirming. However, the baby is not moving less; only the quality of the movement changes.

The best way to reassure yourself that the baby is moving sufficiently is to count fetal movements. Start early in pregnancy at about 25 weeks and continue until delivery so you become familiar with your baby's movement patterns.

Because high blood glucose levels seem to stimulate the baby, the best time of day to count fetal movements is right after eating lunch or dinner. Lie down on your left side. Using a clock with a second hand, time how long it takes your baby to move at least 10 times. Babies usually have 20-minute sleep cycles every hour, so if your baby doesn't move right away, don't be alarmed. If after 1 hour you don't feel movement at least 10 times, count for another hour. On the other hand, if your baby moves 10 times in the first 10 or 15 minutes, then you are done. You don't need to count anymore.

If you do not feel the baby move at least 10 times in 2 hours, call your health care provider. He or she may want you to be monitored to be sure that your baby is okay. Check with your provider to find out what the specific recommendations are regarding the occurrence of fetal movements.

Counting fetal movements is something that you can do every day. In addition to becoming more aware of your baby, lying on your left side for an hour or so every day will help increase blood flow to your baby and give you the rest that your body needs during this very special time of your life.

Understanding Premature Labor

Premature labor is labor that occurs more than three weeks before a woman is expected to deliver. The uterus starts to contract, causing the cervix (opening to the uterus) to open earlier than normal. This can result in the birth of a premature baby.

Unless a woman has experienced premature labor in the past, it is hard to predict who is at risk for premature labor. It can happen to anyone. Recent research suggests that maternal dehydration, urinary tract infections, and motionless standing for long periods may predispose a pregnant woman to premature labor. Women who are pregant with twins, triplets, or more are also at a greater risk. Other than staying well-hydrated, moving around, and monitoring signs of infections, at this time the best way to prevent a baby from being born prematurely is to be alert to warning signs.

Premature labor is usually not painful, which is why many women don't even realize that premature labor is occurring. The following warning signs warrant immediate attention from your obstetrical health care provider.

   Uterine contractions. A contraction is a tightening of the uterus that happens regularly every 5 to 10 minutes for 1 hour (more than 5 contractions in an hour). The uterus is a muscle just like the muscle in your arm. Flex your biceps muscle and feel the difference between a contracting muscle and a relaxed muscle. After 20 weeks of pregnancy, feel your uterus at least once a day for a 20-minute period. Braxton Hicks contractions will be irregular and do not cause the cervix to open.

   Menstrual-like cramps. These cramps may come and go or be consistent.

   Low, dull backache. The backache may come and go or be consistent.

   Pelvic pressure. It will feel as though the baby is pushing down. Women may feel heaviness in the lower abdomen, back, or thighs. The pressure may be consistent or come and go.

▪ Abdominal cramping. This cramping may or may not be accompanied by diarrhea.

▪ Sudden increase in vaginal discharge. The discharge may be mucousy, watery, or lightly bloody.

Making Love During Pregnancy

Now that you are feeling more energetic and the nausea has most likely subsided, you might want to think about your relationship with your partner. Making love is more than just the physical act. Many couples enjoy great satisfaction from just cuddling and being with each other. After all, there are two of you to cuddle now! A good sex life enhances your immune function, elevates your mood, decreases stress, and is an important part of keeping your mind and body in optimal health.

Make time to be with your partner in all aspects of your life—physically, mentally, and emotionally. It is easy to be so consumed with your pregnancy, you forget how you got this way in the first place. Talk with your partner and explore how he is feeling during all this pregnancy stuff! Acknowledge his feelings and discuss any areas of concern.

It is especially important now to create positive communication patterns that are nurturing, understanding, and not judgmental. Make a pact with your partner that you will not belittle his feelings if he doesn't belittle yours. If you don't already have it, try to create an atmosphere of mutual respect for each other's wants, needs, and concerns. The better relationship you have with your partner before the baby arrives, the easier it will be to get through the early days postpartum when you have a new member of the family in the house and stress can be high.

Be clear with your partner about expectations you have regarding help with the baby and around the house. Also listen to your partner's expectations. Be empathetic about his needs. His body is not undergoing changes throughout the pregnancy, but he is still deeply affected mentally and emotionally. Men sometimes even develop "sympathy bellies," especially if they try to eat the same amount of food as their pregnant partners!

Sex is an important part of a relationship. While you are talking about everything else, discuss your sexual relationship and how it has or has not been altered by this pregnancy. You don't have to worry that intercourse will hurt the baby or that the penis will somehow come in contact with the baby. The amniotic sac and the thick mucous plug in the cervix help protect the baby from the outside world.

Discuss sexual concerns with your obstetrical health care provider. If for some reason you are not allowed to have intercourse (for example, because of preterm labor, placenta previa, infection, or bleeding), there are other ways to express love and affection for your partner.

The belly has grown larger in the second trimester, which may present a challenge when using the positions you prefer during lovemaking. Here are several common alternatives to the missionary position:

- Lying on the side. Lie on your side next to your partner, facing the same direction.
- Man behind. Use the bed to support your upper body.
- Woman on top.

The greatest gift you can give your new baby is loving parents who know how to communicate in positive ways. If you sense any problems in your relationship with the baby's father, now is the time to work them out. Care enough about your baby to seek help if you need it!

chapter **9**

Staying Positive in the Third Trimester

Pessimism is bad for your health! When you are sad or stressed or think negative thoughts, hormones are secreted that constrict blood flow to your internal organs as well as your baby, increase your blood pressure, and decrease immune function, making you more vulnerable to fatigue and illness. In labor, pessimism may contribute to slowing down the eventual birth of your baby.

Thinking Positively

In addition to regular exercise, good nutrition and practicing relaxation breathing, learning ways to think positively can help you cope more effectively with labor and delivery and lift your spirits throughout the entire childbirth experience. Here are some suggestions for thinking positively during childbirth and beyond:

Look for lessons. When something happens that makes you sad, instead of wondering, *Why me?* ask yourself, *What I am supposed to learn?* Then listen to your mind and heart for the answer. Try to figure out what is to be gained by having this experience.

Choose to be happy. When you think negative thoughts, force yourself to think about something that makes you feel good. For example, if you make a mistake, instead of beating yourself up think about the times that you did something really well. Make a list of all things you like about yourself.

Be good to yourself. Write down everything that brings you pleasure. Then make a point of trying to do at least one thing on your list each day. Some people think that taking time for themselves is a waste, but when you feel good about yourself, you actually become more efficient.

Stick with realistic goals. When you succeed at something, you feel good about yourself. If you are unable to meet your deadlines or objectives, change your goals so they are more realistic. Instead of giving yourself vague goals such as "clean the garage," break tasks into smaller objectives such as "put tools away" or "organize hoses." Keep to-do lists and prioritize. Cross out those things you finish as you go along to gain a sense of accomplishment.

Remember, it can always be worse. When you are feeling sad or depressed, think of someone who is even less lucky than you to gain a new perspective and possibly come up with ideas on how to cope.

Exercising With a Chair

Now that you are in your last trimester of pregnancy, you may find some of the exercises you were doing before no longer comfortable. Many women have difficulty sitting on the floor for extended periods in the last trimester. Also, the increased weight and size of the baby may interfere with your ability to perform certain exercises. Using a chair when you exercise may help you feel better without putting excess stress on your body.

Question: My back aches when I am sitting. What exercises will help me feel better?

Answer: When the abdominal muscles tire, the back takes over. When sitting, use good back support either on a chair or leaning against a wall. To soothe an aching back, these exercises may help:

- For the rounded cat stretch (see figure 1.2, page 6), begin in table-top position. Exhale and tilt the pelvis forward, rounding the back. Inhale and return the back to the tabletop position.

- For the hip stretch, sit with the knees bent and the soles of the feet together. Reach the hands toward your feet while keeping your back straight. Feel the stretch in your hips. Release forward when you can't go any further. Hold the stretch for 3 to 5 breaths and then slowly roll up the spine with the shoulders and head coming up last.

- For the garland pose (see figure 1.14, page 16), breathe normally while reaching forward. Try to get the heels on the floor. Stay in this position for 3 to 5 breaths.

- Try the squatting pose (see figure 1.11, page 14). Stay in this position for 3 to 5 breaths.

Some of the strengthening exercises in this chapter have counterstretches to help maintain muscle integrity as well as decrease risk of injury. It is important not to skip these complementary stretches.

Posture and Breathing

Sit on the edge of the chair with your back straight and your knees bent at a 90-degree angle. Keep the arms relaxed by your sides and the shoulders comfortably pressed down the back (figure 9.1). Practice belly breathing as described in chapter 3 (page 47).

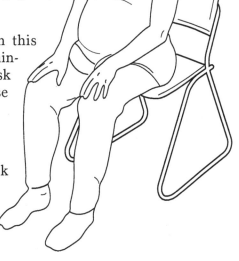

FIGURE 9.1   Chair posture and breathing.

Neck Stretches

Sit on a chair in good posture. As you exhale, bend the head forward and breathe into the back of the neck. Keep the back straight and focus on bringing the chin toward the chest. Inhale and bring the head back on top of the shoulders. Exhale and bring the right ear toward the right shoulder (figure 9.2a). Breathe into the side of the neck. Hold the position for 3 to 5 breaths, then inhale and bring the head up. On the next exhalation, bring the left ear to the left shoulder. Hold the position for 3 to 5 breaths, then lift the head as you inhale.

Inhale and look up at the ceiling. Feel the stretch in the front of the neck. Slowly open and close your mouth for 3 to 5 breaths (figure 9.2b). Inhale and return the head to the starting position.

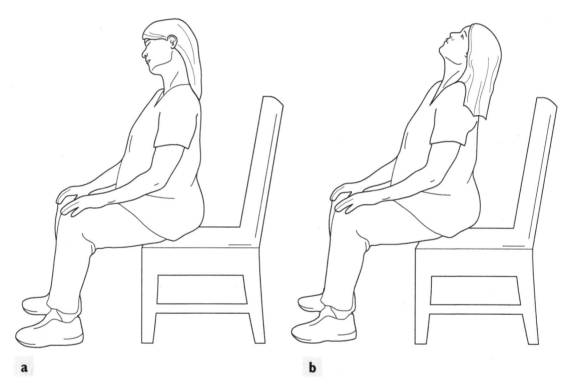

a   b

FIGURE 9.2   **Neck stretch:** *(a)* **bring the right ear to the right shoulder;** *(b)* **look at the ceiling and open your mouth.**

Imagine a piece of chalk at the end of your nose. Pretend to draw a circle on an imaginary blackboard in front of you. Continue for 3 to 5 breaths and then reverse the circle. You can also draw figure eights in both directions.

Shoulder Stretches

Inhale and bring the shoulders up to the ears. Exhale and slide the shoulders down and back. Repeat this movement for 3 to 5 breaths. Circle the shoulders forward 3 to 5 times and then backward 3 to 5 times.

Torso Stretches

For the rib cage isolation, extend the arms out to the sides at shoulder level. Inhale while reaching the arms over to the right (figure 9.3a). Exhale and return to center. Inhale and reach the arms to the left. Exhale and return to center. Repeat the exercise 4 times, alternating right and left sides.

For side stretches, inhale and bring your left arm up toward the left ear, keeping the right arm relaxed by your side. Exhale and bend the torso toward the right (figure 9.3b). Hold the position for 2 to 3 breaths. Inhale and return to center. Repeat the exercise on the opposite side.

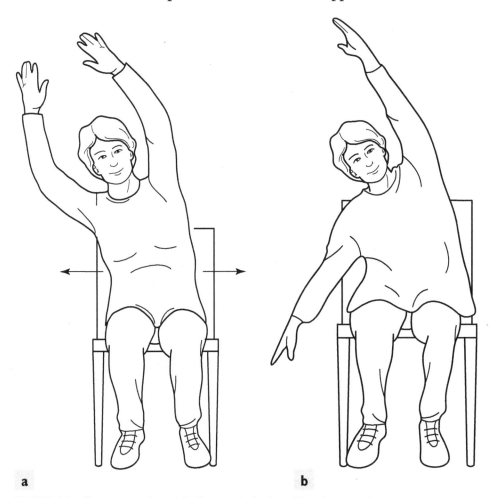

a   b

FIGURE 9.3 Torso stretches: *(a)* rib cage isolation; *(b)* side stretches.

Hip Stretches

For the forward stretch, separate your knees a little more than hip-width apart and relax your hands on top of your knees. Keeping the back straight, bend forward at the hips to bring your torso toward your knees. Allow the hands to slide down the front of your shins (figure 9.4). When you can't go any further, release the back. Relax for 3 to 5 breaths and then slowly roll up the spine, returning to the center. Repeat the stretch 2 to 3 more times.

Then, slowly circle the hips in one direction twice and then in the other direction twice.

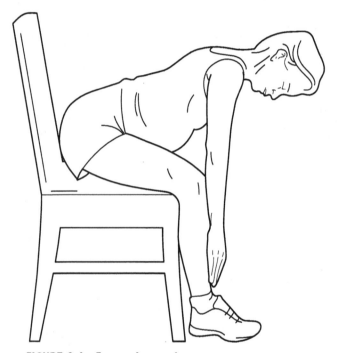

FIGURE 9.4   Forward stretch.

Question: The pressure in my pubic area is very uncomfortable. Are there exercises that will help?

Answer: As the baby grows and starts to descend into the pelvis, you may feel the pressure in your pubic area. Here are two exercises that might help bring relief:

- For the bound angle (see figure 5.9, page 87), sit in good posture with the soles of the feet together and hands wrapped around the ankles or feet. Breathe deeply while concentrating on reaching the knees toward the floor and lifting the spine out of the pelvis. Stay in this position for 3 to 5 breaths.

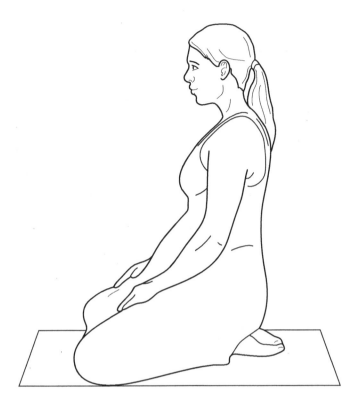

- For the frog pose, sit on the heels and separate the knees as far as you comfortably can while keeping your big toes touching each other (see the illustration). Use the arms to stabilize the upper body. Try to tuck the pelvis under and bring the hips in front of the heels. Sit in this position for 3 to 5 breaths.

Leg and Calf Stretches

To practice the single-leg stretch, extend one leg in front while keeping the other leg bent. Flex the foot of the extended leg. Interlace the fingers on top of the opposite leg (figure 9.5a). While exhaling, keep your back straight and bend forward. Stay in this position for 3 to 5 breaths. Inhale and return to center. Repeat the exercise on the other side.

For foot flexion and extension, sit in good posture. Extend one leg in front. Flex the foot of the extended leg toward your head and hold for 1 to 2 breaths (figure 9.5b). Extend the ball of the foot forward while keeping the toes relaxed. Hold the position for 1 to 2 breaths. Repeat the sequence 8 to 10 times.

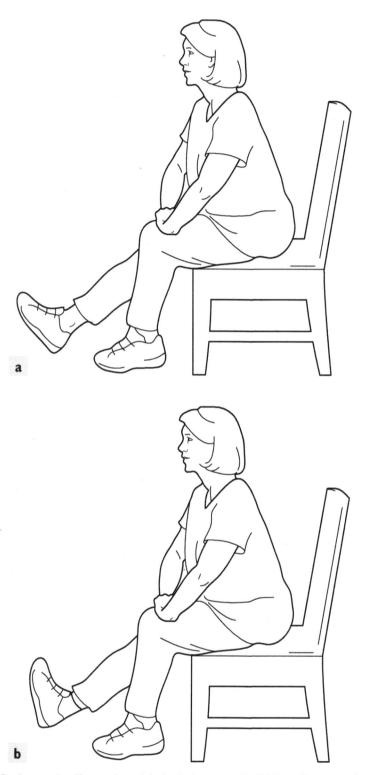

FIGURE 9.5   Leg and calf stretches: *(a)* single-leg stretch; *(b)* foot flexion and extension.

Question: Could you suggest exercises for swollen ankles?

Answer: Lie on your side and extend one leg away from the body. Slowly rotate the ankle in one direction and then in the other direction. Bend your knee and hold the ankle with the hand of the same side and feel the stretch in the front of the thigh and hip flexor muscle (refer to quadriceps stretch on page 85). Then bring your knee up toward your shoulder and hold with the arm of the same side. Extend the leg up to the ceiling and hold with the same arm (see illustration below). Breathe into the stretch for 3 to 5 breaths and return the leg to the floor. Repeat the exercise on the other side.

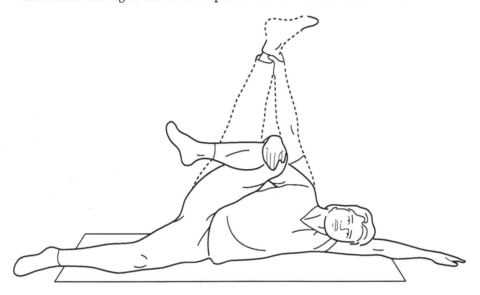

Swimming is also a great way to reduce ankle swelling. If you don't have access to a pool, fill the bathtub with warm water and sit with the water up to your neck for at least 20 minutes. The pressure of the water on your body may help reduce ankle swelling.

Abdominal and Back Strengtheners

For the sitting cat stretch, exhale, hugging your baby with your abdomen, and tilting forward at the hips. Round the lower back (figure 9.6a). As you inhale, start at the base of the spine and slowly straighten your back. Repeat the stretch a total of 8 to 10 times and try to practice twice a day. Integrate Kegels if you can by tightening your pelvic floor as you hug your baby with your abdomen.

FIGURE 9.6a   Sitting cat stretch.

For the standing cat stretch, stand with the feet hip-width apart, the knees bent to about a 45-degree angle and the hands comfortably resting on top of the knees. Keep the back straight and the knees over the ankles. As you exhale, hug your baby with your abdomen and round the lower back, tilting the hips forward (figure 9.6b). As you inhale, start at the base of the spine and slowly straighten your back. Repeat the stretch a total of 8 to 10 times.

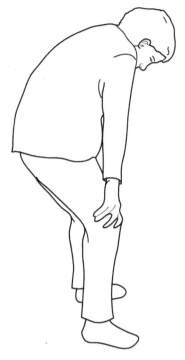

FIGURE 9.6b   **Standing cat stretch.**

Torso rotations strengthen the muscles that rotate the trunk. Sit in correct posture and bring the arms up to the sides at shoulder level. Exhale and rotate the torso to the right (figure 9.6c). Take a breath and exhale, bringing the left hand toward the right knee, making a C shape with your torso. Inhale while straightening your back and then exhale and return to center. Repeat the exercise on the other side. Alternate sides for a total of 8 to 10 times on each side.

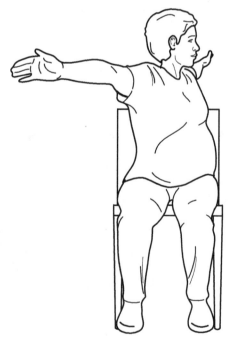

FIGURE 9.6c   **Torso rotations.**

For arm and leg extensions, stand on the side of a chair. Place both hands on the seat and keep the back straight with the knees slightly bent. While breathing normally, extend the right arm beside the right ear and lift the left leg behind you (figure 9.6d). Hold the position for 3 to 5 breaths. Repeat the exercise on the other side and then follow with either a sitting or standing cat stretch.

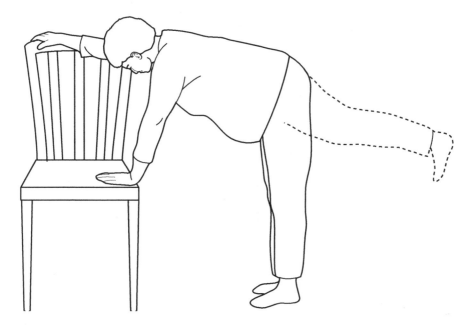

FIGURE 9.6d *Arm and leg extensions.*

Hip and Buttock Strengtheners

For leg circles, stand to the side of a chair, holding it with your hand. Stay in good posture while circling your outside leg at the hip joint in one direction for 3 to 5 breaths (figure 9.7a). Reverse the direction. Move to the other side of the chair and repeat with other leg. Circle the leg in both directions. Then perform the counterstretch: Sit with one leg resting on the other with the knee bent. As you exhale, lean your body forward to stretch out the hip (figure 9.7b). Stay in this posture for 3 to 5 breaths, then change sides.

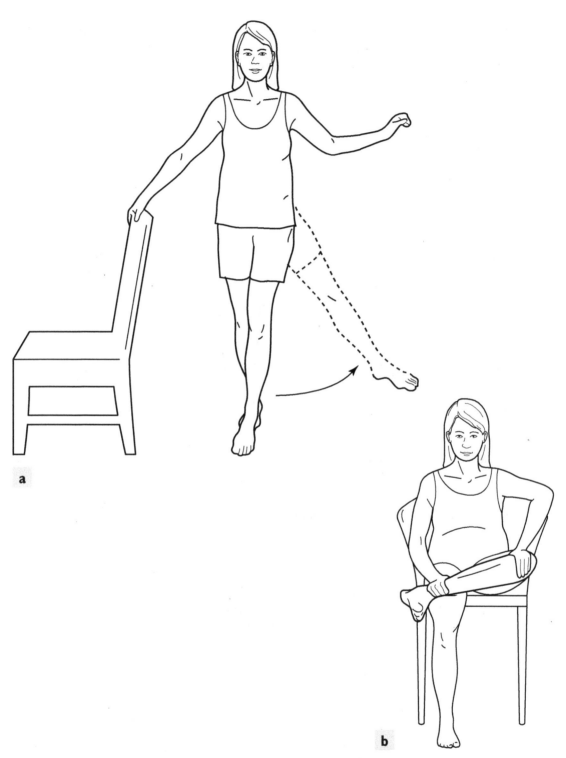

FIGURE 9.7 Leg circles: *(a)* circle the right leg; *(b)* counterstretch by leaning forward to stretch out the hip.

To perform buttock lifts, sit on the edge of the chair with your hands on both sides. As you exhale, squeeze your buttocks, tilt hips forward, and lift your seat (if you can) slightly off the chair (figure 9.8a). Inhale and return to the chair. Repeat 8 to 10 times. Then perform the counterstretch: Stand in front of your chair and hold the seat with both arms, and your legs a little wider than hip-width apart. Keeping your back straight, slowly bend your knees into a squat position while shifting your weight onto your heels (figure 9.8b). Stay in this position for 3 to 5 breaths.

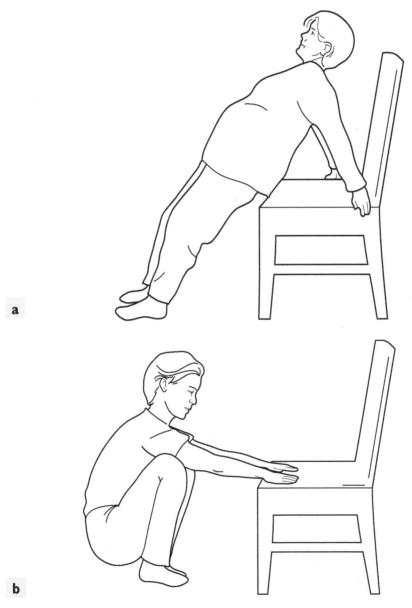

a

b

FIGURE 9.8 Buttock lifts: *(a)* lift slightly off the chair; *(b)* counterstretch by squatting.

Arm Strengtheners

If getting on the mat to do cat bows is too uncomfortable now, practice cat bows on the chair. Stand facing your chair and bring the arms to the seat, with the knees slightly bent and the back straight. As you inhale, bend the elbows and lower the chest toward the chair. Exhale and straighten the arms (figure 9.9a). Repeat the exercise 8 to 10 times. Then perform the counterstretch: Reach behind your back with both hands. Interlace the fingers and bring the palms together (figure 9.9b). Keep the shoulders integrated into your upper back and hold the position for 3 to 5 breaths.

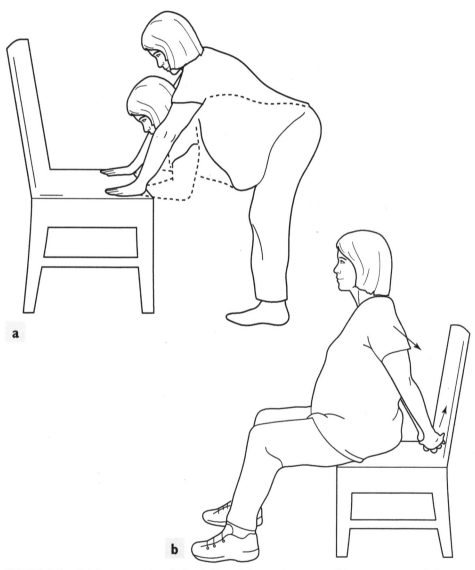

FIGURE 9.9 Cat bows on the chair: *(a)* straighten the arms; *(b)* counterstretch by bringing the palms together behind your back.

For arm extensions, start with the arms out to your sides at shoulder level and the palms turned forward. Exhale and bend the elbows. Bring the hands toward the chest (figure 9.10a). Keep the elbows at or slightly below the shoulders. Inhale and turn the palms so they face forward again. Extend the arms out to the sides while squeezing the shoulder blades together and moving the arms slightly beyond the shoulders (figure 9.10b). Repeat the sequence 8 to 10 times.

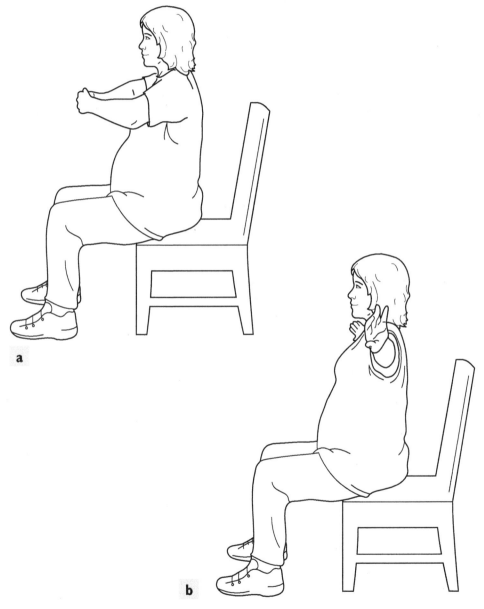

FIGURE 9.10   Arm extensions: (a) bring the hands to the chest; (b) move the arms beyond the shoulders.

Sciatica in Pregnancy

Sciatica is defined as pain along one or both of the sciatic nerves that extend from the lower part of the spinal cord down the legs to the feet. Symptoms may also include a tingling or numbness sensation running down the buttock, hip, and thigh.

In individuals who are not pregnant, the most common cause of sciatica is a herniated disc that presses on one of the nerve roots. However, during the latter months of pregnancy, sciatica is usually caused by the pressure of the pregnant uterus on the sciatic nerve or the baby pressing on the sciatic nerve. In most cases, sciatic pain during pregnancy is not a cause for concern, but it is advisable to inform your obstetrical health provider, who can detect if a more serious condition exists.

In addition to taking warm baths and using a heating pad or cold pack (try both and see which one feels the best), following these tips may also give you relief:

Sleep and rest on the side opposite the side that is bothering you. This may help move the baby or your uterus away from your affected sciatic nerve.

Question: Every time I lie on my side to exercise, I get terrible heartburn. Any suggestions?

Answer: Heartburn in the third trimester is usually associated with the baby pressing on the diaphragm. When you lie down, the pressure increases, causing reflux of stomach contents into the esophagus. Try eating something light, such as a piece of fruit or yogurt, more than two hours before exercise. Also, use a pillow to lift your head above your stomach. This may help to prevent reflux.

Rest in a knee–chest position as often as possible (figure 9.11). You may also rest your head and upper body on a pillow for added comfort.

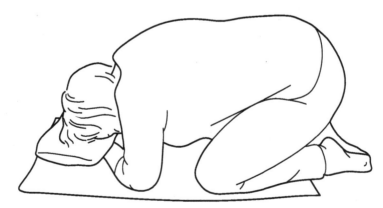

FIGURE 9.11   Knee–chest position.

Perform pelvic tilts while lying on your side (figure 9.12) or from a table-top position. As you exhale, tilt your hips forward and round your back into a rounded cat stretch. Return to a tabletop position while inhaling. Gently move your back from tabletop to a rounded cat stretch, coordinating movements with your breath. Perform this exercise 5 times, several times a day. Stop exercising if you experience any pain.

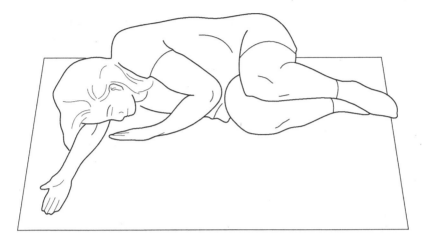

FIGURE 9.12   Sidelying pelvic tilts.

Pros and Cons of Episiotomy

An episiotomy is an incision made in the perineum by an obstetrical health care provider to widen the opening of the birth canal to allow more room for the baby to pass through. The perineum is the area of skin between the vagina (birth canal) and the anus. Episiotomies are used in about 60 percent of deliveries in the United States.

Many obstetrical health care providers believe that episiotomies help prevent tearing of the skin and the vaginal lining during birth. The idea is that a precise incision is easier to repair and takes less time to heal than a natural tear in the skin. Women most likely to have an episiotomy are first-time moms, are having large babies, or are delivering breech babies.

In the early to mid-1900s, anesthesia that was commonly used for childbirth made women disoriented and unable to push effectively. Many babies were delivered using forceps, which helped pull the baby from the birth canal. Episiotomies became routine procedures to avoid tearing the perineum during forceps deliveries. Unfortunately, an episiotomy incision may cause excessive bleeding or may tear into the rectum. As unmedicated childbirth became more popular in the 1970s, many people criticized the use of episiotomies as a routine procedure.

For women who want to avoid an episiotomy, daily massages of the perineum are recommended during the last six weeks of pregnancy. While perineal massage may help prevent an episiotomy, it is not a guarantee. Your obstetrical health care provider will have to make many last-minute decisions to do what's best for you and your baby.

Some circumstances arise that necessitate an episiotomy. Discuss your feelings about an episiotomy with your obstetrical care provider. The ultimate decision on whether or not to have any episiotomy, however, is best made by your experienced provider during the delivery process.

Perineal Massage

The perineum is the triangular layer of skin between the vagina and the anus in females and between the scrotum and anus in males. Beneath the perineum in females are the muscles and fibrous tissues that stretch to accommodate the baby during childbirth.

Historically, physicians believed that episiotomies would help decrease the risk of vaginal lacerations and perineal tears during childbirth. (An episiotomy is an incision made into the perineum at the end of the second stage of labor to help facilitate the birth of the baby.) However, research during the 1970s and 1980s revealed that not only have episiotomies failed to prevent lacerations and perineal tears, they actually tend to increase the incidence and severity of lacerations associated with childbirth. Since then, researchers have been studying other variables that might decrease the incidence and severity of vaginal lacerations and perineal tears. Three variables have been identified, including maternal position, style of pushing, and perineal massage.

From 1979 to 1985, researchers in the northwestern part of the United States studied 368 women whose deliveries had been attended to by a home-based midwifery practice. The women were primarily white with 61 first-time moms (primiparas) and 307 women who had already birthed at least one other child (multiparas).

Even though findings indicated that first time moms had more vaginal lacerations than multiparous women, the severity of lacerations were less serious in women who practiced perineal massage. Multiparous women who had received episiotomies for previous deliveries were also found to derive benefits from performing perineal massage this time around.

Although there are still questions concerning the optimum frequency, timing, and technique of perineal massage, researchers encourage pregnant women to practice it to help prevent or decrease the severity of vaginal lacerations and perineal tears associated with childbirth. This type of massage helps women prepare for the stretching sensation during the birth of a baby as well as reducing the need for episiotomy and risk of perineal tearing.

Start daily perineal massage around 34 weeks of pregnancy. Be sure to discuss perineal massage with your obstetrical health care provider before practicing this technique. Partners can also be taught to perform perineal massage. Avoid perineal massage if you have any active vaginal infections, including herpes.

Wash your hands. Find a comfortable, warm, private place to practice. Position a mirror in front of your perineum to see what you are doing. Lubricate your fingers and perineum with vegetable oil, cocoa butter, water-based lubricating jelly, or vitamin E oil.

Place the thumbs inside the vagina about 1 to 1 1/2 inches and press down and to the sides to gently stretch the skin. This might cause a slight tingling or burning sensation. Avoid moving upward toward the urethra. Hold a steady pressure for about two minutes until the perineum starts to feel numb.

Gently massage the oil into the lower half of the vagina for another couple of minutes while pulling down and outward with the thumbs. This motion simulates the way the perineal skin will be stretched during childbirth.

Making a Birth Plan

Every pregnant woman dreams of her fantasy labor. It's a way of coping with an event that is unknown and a little overwhelming. In most cases, labor and delivery are very different than the fantasy. Regardless, it is still a good idea to develop a birth plan according to your personal preferences. This gives your provider important information that may influence the course of your labor. First, look for things you can control.

Serenity Prayer

Give us serenity to accept what cannot be changed, courage to change what should be changed, and wisdom to know the one from the other.

—*14th Century*

Things You Can Control

When you plan your labor, think about what you need to bring to the hospital and start to get those things ready. Pack two bags, one to go with you to labor and the other that could be brought in after you deliver.

In your labor bag, place your favorite music and a battery operated audiocassette or CD player. Include an object such as a picture to use as a focal point. Be sure to include a camera, film, and batteries. Bring a list of important phone numbers and either a portable phone or change for a pay phone. Be sure to include your insurance cards, ID, and any hospital registration papers. Bring lollipops or hard candy because your mouth may get dry during labor.

Also, bring your glasses if you wear contact lenses and leave the contacts at home. When you are in labor, your eyes will get tired and dry. In addition, if for some reason you need to have a cesarean, you would not be allowed to wear your contact lenses. The less you bring with you to the hospital, the less risk of losing valuable items. So, refrain from wearing jewelry with the exception of your wedding band if you wear one.

In your suitcase, include a nightgown to wear a day or two after delivery. Plan to wear the hospital gown most of the time while you are in the hospital. It makes more sense to get the hospital gown dirty rather than one of your nightgowns. Also pack your bathrobe, socks, and slippers. Try to remember to bring your baby book and ask the nurses to footprint your baby's feet right in the book if there is a space designated. If you are planning to nurse, purchase a gown with slits for that purpose. Many women put on the nightgown when they have company and then wear a hospital gown the rest of the time.

Include personal care items such as your toothbrush, toothpaste, facial cleanser, moisturizer, nursing pads, perineal pads, and makeup in your suitcase. Bring a supportive bra or a nursing bra if you will be nursing. Bring your own pillow if you think you would like to have it.

You probably will not fit into your regular clothes by the time you go home, so be sure to bring maternity clothes or loose-fitting clothes to go home in. Typically, your belly will be swollen the first couple of days after delivery. Plan on it!

Bring clothes for the baby to wear to go home. Bring a small cap regardless of the weather. Even in warm weather, there might be a concern about air conditioning in the car and house. Babies lose most of their heat through the top of the head. Bring anything else you feel is important to create a safe, positive space for you and your baby.

The tools you have learned throughout your pregnancy will be the most help for you during labor and delivery. Tools such as breathing, relaxation, exercising, and meditation will come into play during labor and delivery. All of these tools will assist you and can be used anytime, anywhere.

If, however, you find these tools not to be working, you do have a choice of whether or not to receive pain relief medication. Even if you think you do not want to be medicated, talk to your provider about what is available to you. This way, if you decide later to have medication, you will already know your choices.

Once you are in labor, decisions of this nature are hard to make. Include your partner in conversations with your provider. He should support whatever decisions you make and understand that his role is to support you, not tell you what to do.

If you are doing well and your baby is doing well, ask to walk around as much as you can. Gravity can actually help labor progress. You may also ask for ice chips and sips of water. If you think there are too many people in your room or the room is too hot or cold, have your coach or support person talk to the staff. Helping you to control external distractions is part of the coach's job.

Other choices you should discuss with your health care provider include:

- Laboring or delivering your baby in a tub
- Taking a shower during labor
- Using a birthing bed or chair
- Laboring on a birthing ball
- Constant or intermittent fetal monitoring
- A mirror to watch the birth
- Music during labor
- For you or your partner to cut the cord
- To hold your infant (skin-to-skin contact) and breast-feed right after birth
- Important people that you want in your labor room
- To circumcise or not to circumcise your infant boy

Things You Cannot Control

The best laid plans . . . Too often, situations arise in labor that necessitate a change in plans. An example is if the baby turns out to be breech, feet or butt first. In this situation, most practitioners will recommend a cesarean section. This is a decision made in the best interest of you and your baby. So, how your baby is delivered is basically up to your obstetrical health care provider. You have hopefully chosen a provider who will make decisions in your best interest.

The duration of your labor is not something that anyone can control totally. If you find that your labor is long, and there is no reason to speed it up (for example, the baby is doing well), take the opportunity between contractions to rest. Do not try to rush the labor experience. Babies usually come at their own time. Follow the rhythm of your body and the baby's body. If, however, there are any signs of distress, then turn the decisions over to your provider.

Discuss with your provider your choices regarding monitoring the baby. Every practitioner has different preferences. If you feel differently about monitoring than your provider, discuss your differences before you go into labor. Remember, the goal of labor is not to fulfill all of your fantasies but to have a healthy baby. In some cases, you can achieve both, but in many cases, there will be some things you'll just have to accept.

Expect the Unexpected

How close reality comes to your expectations has everything to do with how well you adjust to the postpartum experience physically, mentally, and emotionally. Even in the best of circumstances, plans need to change. If nothing else, plan to be flexible and you won't be disappointed. No one can predict your labor experience.

Unknowns are difficult to accept. But the more you can go with the flow, the better the chance that you will have a positive childbirth experience. Choose to believe that everything will happen for the best and trust that your body knows what it needs to do.

Labor and delivery will challenge your ability to balance effort and surrender. You need to learn to surrender to each contraction until you finally use all of your effort to push your baby out!

During your daily stretching regimen, practice breathing into tight muscles. Take a breath and feel the lungs expand along with every muscle in your body. As you exhale, feel the tension from your muscles leaving with the breath.

The more accurate you can become in identifying the difference between tension and release in your body, the better able you will be to control your reaction to tension in the hopes of finding release. The more you practice this breathing and relaxation exercise, the more chance this technique will be automatic during your labor. It takes some work, but the results are well worth the effort!

chapter 10

Training for Labor and Delivery

After practicing all of the exercises in this book, including the breathing and relaxation techniques, you should be feeling physically and mentally prepared for the labor and delivery experience. As an athlete trains for an event, the more prepared you are to meet the challenges of childbirth, the easier it will be.

It is hard to prove that exercising during pregnancy will result in an easy labor. There are too many variables affecting both exercise and labor to make any promises. It is evident, though, that fit women are able to handle the task of labor a lot better then women who are not physically or mentally prepared.

Yes, labor is a challenge. But by being strong, stretched, and centered, you will have a rich and rewarding experience.

Discomfort During Labor

Before the 20th century, childbirth was regarded as a natural process requiring a significant amount of effort associated with a bearable level of pain. However, in the United States, there seems to be a belief that labor pain is bad and the laboring woman should be relieved of her pain whenever possible. Some even suggest that abdominal surgery be performed to relieve the pain of labor.

These beliefs seem paradoxical in a society that celebrates individuals who endure great pain and distress in pursuit of mountain peaks or marathon races. Even though labor pain is pain with a purpose, labor is not a competition to see how much pain a woman can tolerate. The concern, however, is that sometimes the type of medication used during labor and the dosages required to control the pain adequately may negatively affect the baby.

There is also evidence that satisfaction with the birthing experience is greater in those women who are able to birth their babies without medication. Just like the athlete who is able to complete the race or marathon despite some physical discomfort, the choice to have a medicated birth is individual and should be discussed between the expectant mom and her health care provider. There are several situations when the benefits of medication outweigh the risks.

Let's first look at the advantages of feeling pain in labor. (Yes, there are advantages to feeling pain!) One theory of why women have pain in labor is to give the expectant mother warning of impending birth. Without some physical warning, a laboring woman would not know when to either get herself to a facility or notify her practitioner.

Every woman's experience of labor is different depending on several variables. An individual's pain threshold plays an important factor in the experience of discomfort and pain during labor as does culture and ethnicity. Labor pain occurs in the context of cultural beliefs, mores, and standards of the family and community as well as the health care system and its providers. Pain behaviors vary greatly among different cultures as a result of learned patterns of expected behavior.

Researchers have found that women who live in rural areas have a more healthful attitude toward birthing than women in urban settings. Growing up around farms, women see animals birthing all the time, so there is no mystery to this naturally occurring event. There is also evidence that having extended family members around during the birth improves outcomes.

Labor pain is also dependent on the different stages of labor. During the first stage of labor (dilatation phase), abdominal pain dominates with pain stimuli arising from the mechanical distention of the lower uterine segment and cervical dilatation.

Typically, the intensity of labor pain increases with greater cervical dilatation, and is positively correlated with the intensity, duration, and frequency of uterine contractions. There are also differences between primiparas (first-time moms) and multiparas (women with more than one previous delivery). First-time moms in early labor (before 5 centimeters dilation) on average experience greater sensory pain than women who have previously delivered a baby. They may also experience an increase in labor pain during descent and the second stage of labor.

Although most women experience lower abdominal pain during contractions, 15 to 74 percent also experience contraction-related lower back pain. Researchers report a significant positive relationship between menstrual-related back pain and back pain during labor. The etiology of this relationship is still not well understood.

Fetal position and the position of the laboring woman can cause back pain during labor. Most women experience more comfort when standing rather than lying flat on the back. Prior experience with non-gynecologic pain may be associated with decreased pain in labor. Belief is that previous experience in handling pain provides an opportunity to develop pain-coping skills. For many first-time moms, childbirth is the first experience of significant physical pain.

Researchers believe that is why women who exercise on a regular basis have a better ability to cope with the pain in labor, because they are accustomed to feeling some muscular discomfort associated with moderate exercise. As with exercise, pain in labor is a temporary discomfort with positive end results.

A woman's confidence in her ability to cope with labor pain has a powerful relationship to decreased pain perception. The success of coping skills learned in a childbirth education class is determined by the woman's belief that she is able to do so.

Whether you think you can or whether you think you can't, you're right.

Mark Twain

Environmental factors influence pain perception during labor. People present at the labor can either help the laboring woman or be a detriment. Verbal and nonverbal communications, philosophy of care, practice policies of providers, quality of support, degree of strangeness of the facility, noise, lighting, and temperature all affect the experience of the laboring woman. How restrictive the environment is in terms of space and ability to move within the space are also important factors.

Helplessness and suffering are experienced when individuals have insufficient resources and are unable to cope. If a woman understands the origin of her pain (cervical dilatation and fetal descent), views the eventual birth as highly positive, and perceives labor and the accompanying pain as a nonthreatening life experience to overcome, she may experience pain but will not suffer. These women are the ones who experience an increase in self-esteem as a result of childbirth.

When a laboring woman is comforted through physical measures, given a safe environment to labor, surrounded by supportive people, and well-prepared with effective coping skills, she tends to be able to better handle the discomfort of labor and delivery and seems to experience a sense of empowerment from the total birthing experience.

Some natural comfort measures can be used to reduce the laboring woman's pain during labor and delivery. They are discussed next.

Relaxation

Relaxation is the number one skill to be learned to decrease your pain and discomfort in labor and delivery. All the other comfort measures and complementary therapies either enhance relaxation or help prevent tension to begin with. Learning to relax prevents stress hormones, called catecholamines, from being released in the first place.

Catecholamines act as constrictors, causing the muscles in the body, including those in the uterus, to tense up. When this happens, the longitudinal muscle fibers work against the inner circular muscle fibers in the uterus, causing considerably more pain and increasing the length of labor.

On the flip side, when you are relaxed, you allow endorphins—the body's natural pain killers—to be released. Endorphins produce a tranquil, amnesiac state and decrease one's perception of pain. Endorphins are released during exercise, and it is partly because of endorphins that marathon runners and triathletes can push themselves to the limits that they do.

Stress is a part of everyday life. We can't control stress in our lives, but we can control our reaction to it. Relaxation is an art that needs to be practiced every day. The better we are able to relax, the easier it is to relax in stressful situations, including labor and delivery. Begin practicing early in pregnancy, and by the time you need to use it in labor and delivery, it will become second nature.

Breathing

In typical Hollywood having-a-baby scenes, Mom is hooked up to IVs, lying on her back, hee-heeing and hoo-hooing contorting her face in many ways. But this does not have to be you. Many women give testimony of hyperventilating and just not getting the fast-paced breathing patterns typically taught in traditional Lamaze classes. Others feel that it actually increases pain perception by increasing tension. And they're right! After taking a deep, cleansing breath at the beginning of each contraction, breathe slowly in and out through your nose throughout the entire contraction. If your nose is stuffed, breathe however you feel comfortable. When it's over, take another deep cleansing breath.

Proper breathing is very important. During a contraction, the baby is receiving very little oxygen, because the blood vessels going to the baby are also contracted. Slow, tranquil breathing together with the deep, cleansing breaths allow more oxygen to reach the baby. Fast-paced heeing and hooing does not. Learning to breathe correctly, though, is like relaxation techniques—it needs to be practiced! And breathing and relaxation go hand-in-hand. Remember, your breath communicates with your muscles. When breathing is fast, muscle tension builds. When breathing is slow, you are telling your muscles to relax.

Visualization

Visualization is just as it sounds, visualizing or picturing an image in your mind that enhances your body's ability to relax. As we learn more and more about the mind–body connection, we are beginning to understand more about how the mind affects the body. Positive images, such as picturing your cervix as a flower blossom that is gradually opening can help the cervix open more quickly. Visualize your cervix as melting and opening. Think of cool colors—blue, green, purple—to help enhance your relaxation.

Focusing on the baby inside of you can be relaxing and motivating at the same time. Try to picture what your baby looks like. Send loving messages to your baby. Talk to your baby. Imagine what labor might be like from the baby's viewpoint.

Because the hospital is an unfamiliar environment to most people, it helps to visualize a special place where you can go, a place where you feel comfortable, safe, and happy. Practice this visualization throughout your pregnancy so you will have a familiar place to go to during your labor, thereby, putting you more at ease.

Water

Whether you're planning on having a water birth or not, water can be a great addition to your repertoire of tools for helping you through the labor and delivery experience. Many women proclaim the wonders of water during their labor and delivery. "I had a natural childbirth and spent the majority of labor in the bathtub," explains Nancy, mother of two. "During each contraction I would sort of float, and my husband would pour water over my tummy."

"It was awesome!" Judith says. "Water is heavenly." Most hospitals will have policies on whether or not the use of the tub or whirlpool is allowed after your water breaks. If it becomes off-limits, then head to the shower. The feeling of the warm water raining down on your abdomen or pounding on your back can be just what the doctor ordered.

Positioning

There are many different positions to be in during labor and delivery (figure 10.1). The main position to avoid is being flat on your back, because this compresses the vena cava and also prevents gravity from assisting in the descent of your baby. It's also uncomfortable if you are having back labor.

■ Lying on one side. This position helps to relax the back and improves blood flow to the baby during labor. Lying on the left side offers optimal circulation for you and your baby, but if this is uncomfortable, try lying on your right side.

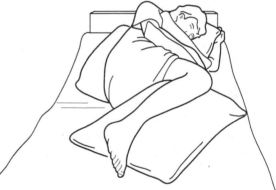

FIGURE 10.1a Lying on one side.

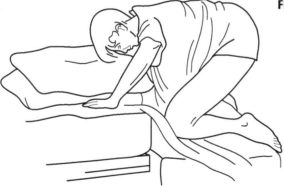

■ Knee-to-chest position. The position is especially good for women experiencing back labor. This position takes the baby off of your back.

FIGURE 10.1b Knee-to-chest position

Squatting with your partner in front. When the baby starts to descend into the pelvis, a lot of pressure is felt on the perineum. Squatting helps relieve discomfort and, with the help of gravity, aids baby in moving down into the birth canal. This can be done with or without a partner, depending on how Mom is feeling.

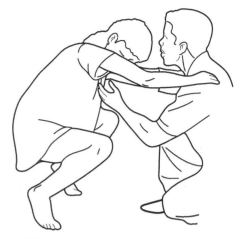

FIGURE 10.1c Squatting with partner in front.

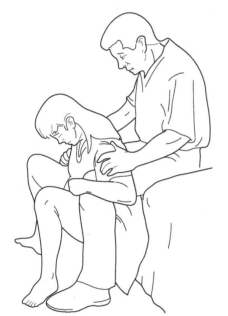

Squatting with your partner behind. If you are unsteady or tired from labor, squatting with the support of a partner behind helps provide more stability and prevents you from falling backward.

FIGURE 10.1d Squatting with partner behind.

Sitting on the edge of a bed. This is another position to help relieve back discomfort. Also, while you are sitting on the bed, your partner is in a perfect position to massage your back. This feels very soothing and nurturing.

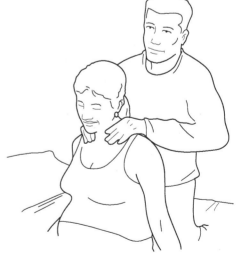

FIGURE 10.1e Sitting on the edge of a bed.

Any of the vertical positions—standing, sitting, leaning over a support, squatting—or the semi-reclined positions utilize gravity. Another popular position is being semi-reclined on the left side. "As far as positions . . . the only one that really worked for me was on my left side with my partner rubbing the bottom of my back with his palm," recalls Carma, mother of three. Like most anything, there are pros and cons to any position. What is important is that it is comfortable to you, and that it is a position in which you are able to concentrate and relax.

When a position becomes uncomfortable, try a new one. Sometimes, though, the change in position can make the next few contractions feel stronger. Give it a few minutes. You will eventually settle in to your new position and come back to your breath.

Exercises to Cope With Labor

Years ago, a researcher in California wanted to study bicycling and its effect on the fetus in labor. He asked one of his patients, who was a professional cyclist, to ride a stationary bike during labor while the baby was being monitored. The result of the study was that riding a bike during labor was in no way harmful to the baby, and in fact, helped to decrease the discomfort of labor.

Exercising during labor may help you better deal with the discomforts of labor as well as help labor progress. Walking is a great way to exercise through labor. It will give you a feeling of well-being as well as allow gravity to help the baby descend into the pelvis naturally. Try each of the following exercises between contractions when labor is progressing normally with no complications.

Shoulder Stretch

Sit comfortably on a chair or floor. Interlace fingers in front of you and turn palms outward (figure 10.2a). Exhale, round the back, and reach the palms forward, flexing at the wrists. Inhale, straighten the back, and reach the arms above your head (figure 10.2b). Separate the hands and bring them behind your back. Interlace your fingers again, bringing the palms together, or grab opposite wrists (figure 10.2c). Pull back on your shoulders as you straighten your arms. Hold the position for 3 to 5 breaths and then release the arms and relax.

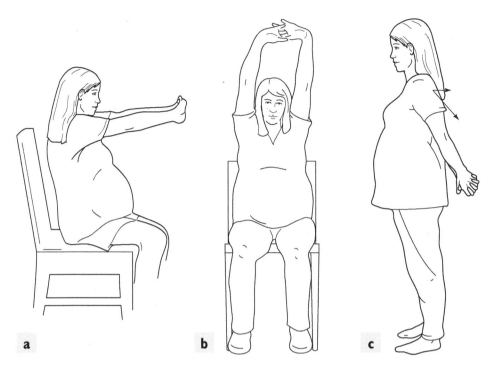

FIGURE 10.2   Shoulder stretch: *(a)* **interlace fingers, palms turned out;** *(b)* **reach the arms above the head;** *(c)* **grab opposite wrists.**

Belly Dance

In ancient times, women would belly dance to prepare the pelvis for childbirth. You can either stand or kneel on all fours in a tabletop position. Start to rotate the pelvis in one direction 3 to 4 times and then reverse the movement in the opposite direction (figure 10.3). If you are standing, keep the knees slightly bent. Be sure to rotate the torso by moving at the hip joints.

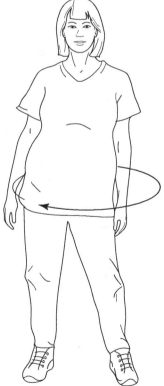

FIGURE 10.3   Belly dance.

Lion Pose

Tighten your face by squeezing your eyes closed and puckering your lips (figure 10.4a). On the exhalation, open your eyes and mouth widely while sticking out your tongue as far as it can go (figure 10.4b). Relax, then do it again. If you want to practice the full pose, when you stick your tongue out, make a roaring sound and lift your eyes upward to look up at the ceiling. This is a great exercise to do when your labor nurse asks how you feel!

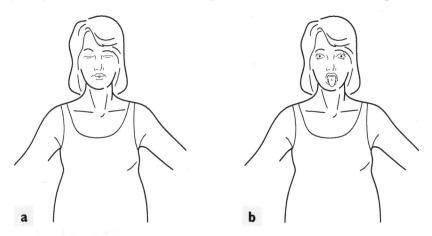

FIGURE 10.4 Lion pose: *(a)* close the eyes and pucker the lips; *(b)* open the eyes and stick out the tongue.

Wall-Assisted Body Stretch

Stand with the feet about 6 inches away from the wall. Place the hands on the wall by leaning forward at the waist. Pull your weight toward your heels and lower the torso toward the floor while keeping the back straight (figure 10.5). Bend your knees if you feel any discomfort in the legs or lower back. Stay in this position for 3 to 5 breaths and then come back up. Repeat this stretch as often as necessary.

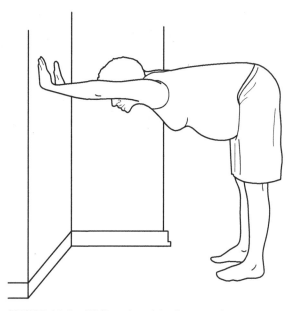

FIGURE 10.5 Wall-assisted body stretch.

Squatting

Sit on your knees on the floor. Move your feet more than hip-width apart and walk your hands toward your knees, rising onto the balls of the feet. Try to bring your weight over the heels and then bring the palms of the hands together in front of your heart with your elbows pressing against the inner aspect of your knees (see figure 1.11, page 14). Sit in this position for 3 to 5 breaths. You can also hold on to a chair or your partner while in this position.

Massage

Massage is one of those comfort measures that everyone seems to have a different opinion on. Pam, mother of two, says that even though she enjoyed massages during her pregnancy, when her husband began rubbing her head and shoulders while she was in labor, "It was really annoying. Mainly I wanted to be left alone so I could maintain focus." For others, the preference for massage is transient. "My husband massaged my stomach and shoulders," says Karen, mother of six, "and stopped when I became touch-sensitive."

Massage and communication go hand-in-hand. At different points in labor, you may want to be touched in different ways. Communicate with your partner and let your wishes be known. Also, let your partner know that you may change your mind frequently and to ask you whether you would like a massage before giving one. What feels good in the beginning may not have the same effect later in labor.

There doesn't have to be any specific method to massage. "If it feels good, do it" is one saying that is very appropriate for this comfort measure. Some massage therapists recommend rubbing the area on the bottom of the foot at the top-center of the pad of the heel (figure 10.6). Because of the cervix–uterine reflex, it is believed that firmly rubbing this area helps alleviate labor pain and also aids in thinning the cervical rim.

Massage is related to other complimentary therapies such as acupressure. Also known as body-work, acupressure involves pressing deeply on certain points on the body to relieve physical symptoms such as pain. Many women have used

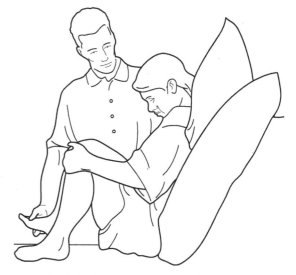

FIGURE 10.6 Foot massage to reduce labor pain.

acupressure to alleviate morning sickness, induce labor, increase relaxation, and decrease labor pain.

Music

Relaxation can be enhanced or hurt by your choice of music during labor and delivery. Some women choose white noise or nature sounds to help them relax. By using these types of audio enhancers, you can choose a visualization that goes along with them. For instance, if you're listening to the sound of a bubbling brook and the chirping sounds of forest wildlife, you can put yourself in that scene.

However, for some people, certain scenarios will not bring peace. At a class I was teaching once, I had an ocean sounds tape. Naturally, it included the distant squawk of seagulls. One of the members sat up straight when the exercise was over and remarked that it did nothing for her because all she could think of was the seagulls who attacked her once on the beach! Choose music that you associate with feelings of calm.

Classical music or CDs and tapes designed specifically for relaxation are great, too. Check with your birthing center to see whether they have a tape or CD player there to use, or if you can bring your own. Also, practice relaxing with the music before labor so you will already have an association between the music and feeling relaxed.

Each birth is as different as each woman who experiences it. Know what tools are available and choose what works for you. Have a plan, but be flexible to changes. Imagine riding the wave of labor as if you were riding a wave in the ocean. There are bumps along the way, but when you go with the flow it will eventually carry you to your destination. Before you know it, you will be the one telling the birth story of your child.

Ready, Get Set, It's Labor Time!

Just as your pregnancy is unlike anyone else's, so will your labor be. Fortunately, though, there are guidelines based on what the average woman will experience. We have not only included the textbook version but also what real women who have been there have to say about birth.

Remember, you can't control what happens to you; you can only control your reaction to it! Giving birth is an experience of letting go. While your uterus works to birth your baby, you need to surrender your control and trust that your body (and your health care provider) will know what to do. By tensing up and resisting contractions, you may actually slow down your labor as well as increase the intensity of the contractions. Hopefully the breathing and meditation exercises you practiced during pregnancy will pay off in the labor and delivery experience.

Stage One: Early and Active Labor

The latent (early) phase of labor begins with the onset of contractions that cause the cervix to soften and open and ends with the onset of active labor. This phase can actually begin weeks before the birth of the baby or it may start and last for 2 to 6 hours.

During this phase, contractions are usually mild and irregular, giving you a pressurelike feeling. Contractions may be anywhere from 5 to 30 minutes apart and 30 to 40 seconds in duration. By the end of this phase, your cervix will have dilated 3 to 4 centimeters.

This is a time in labor when you may feel a lot of mixed emotions. Women report feeling excited, yet nervous and anxious. You may have sensations in your body of pressure in the groin, abdominal cramps, and possibly some back discomfort. But usually in the first phase, women are quite comfortable and can easily breathe through each contraction. This is a good time to rest between contractions to conserve your energy for later.

Question: Is it really possible to relax during a contraction?

Answer: Yes, but it will certainly be difficult to relax during contractions if you have not practiced this skill throughout your pregnancy. You must train your body to do so. During times of stress and anxiety, our bodies release catecholamines. These hormones actually make our pain receptors more receptive to pain, increasing our perception of it. We become more tense, the muscle fibers of the uterus don't work together, and the pain is increased. This is what Dr. Dick Read coined the *fear–tension–pain cycle.* On the other hand, when our bodies and minds are at ease and relaxed, endorphins are released, blocking the pain receptors. The layers of muscle fibers in our uterus can work the way they should, and the cervix can open with less pain and resistance.

Here are some suggestions for getting through the first phase of labor:

- Count contractions. Start timing at the beginning of one contraction and time to the beginning of the next.
- Practice relaxation methods.
- Finish last-minute preparations.
- Rest or take a nap.
- Talk to the baby.
- Eat lightly if you feel hungry.
- Drink lots of fluids.
- Take a walk.
- Take a shower.

Your coach can help you by supporting you and staying calm. Practice relaxation techniques together so your coach won't be overly anxious either. The coach can help with last-minute preparations and talk to the baby, too. The coach can practice timing contractions with Mom.

Women have different things to say about the early phase of labor. Karen says, "I was sleeping when I woke up to crampy labor. The real clue was losing my mucous plug. The contractions become more regular and all-around, but no real pain."

Carma was sleeping as well. "I was sleeping when my labor started with both of my first two pregnancies. I woke up with pains in my back and felt like I had to pee really bad."

"Early labor wasn't painful for me," Marnie says. "My very extended tummy, at 12 days overdue, just felt like it was clenching and releasing, the same way your arm feels when you clench your fist and let it go again."

Question: When should I head to the hospital?

Answer: Your health care provider will tell you, but it's usually when you've had contractions 5 minutes apart for about an hour. However, there are many factors that come into play, including individual differences, distance to the hospital, and whether or not this is your first child. Rule of thumb: If you're uncomfortable being at home, then at least go and have your progress checked out.

The early active phase begins with the onset of active labor and ends at 7 centimeters dilation. The beginning of the transition phase can last 2 to 3 1/2 hours. Contractions are usually moderate to strong and become more regular, arriving 3 to 4 minutes apart and lasting 40 to 60 seconds.

Initially, you may feel very relaxed and comfortable. But with the increasing intensity of contractions, fatigue usually sets in and then you may find yourself becoming irritable and unfocused. This is a good time to refocus your attention during your contractions on something in the room or a picture or object that you like to look at. If you have other children or a special child in your life, ask them to draw or paint you a picture early in your pregnancy that you can focus on during labor.

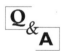

Question: I've heard that I should keep my eyes open and focus on an object during a contraction. But it's more comfortable to me to keep them closed. Am I doing it wrong?

Answer: Absolutely not! Although there are some childbirth education programs that almost insist on the mother keeping her eyes open, you must do what comes naturally to you. It certainly is easier to practice visualization with them shut. Just make sure that when your eyes are closed, you don't squeeze them. Remember to do your body check; the muscles around the eyes should be relaxed.

In this phase, there is usually an increase in bloody show and you may feel achy in your legs, back, and groin. In this phase, your membranes may rupture if they haven't already. Here are some suggestions for getting through the early active phase:

- Continue to focus and practice relaxation and visualization methods right through contractions.
- Stay hydrated by sipping on clear fluids or sucking on ice chips.
- Continue relaxation breathing.
- Urinate frequently.
- Change to whatever position is most comfortable for you.
- Practice the stretching exercises discussed at the beginning of this chapter.
- Keep a positive attitude!

Your coach can help by supporting you. The coach may suggest different positions if you seem uncertain about what to do. The coach needs to listen to what you want and need. The coach might offer fluids and ice chips or a massage. The coach needs to make sure the environment is one that is conducive to relaxation and birth (environmental control).

Women have different experiences in this phase of labor as well. "All my labors felt as if someone was squeezing my stomach and pushing on my back at the same time," says Kathy.

"Third child, all natural," says Roberta. "Absolutely the best experience. Pain, yes, but I worked on focusing and dilating. I brought music with me. I had my friend, as well as my husband. I walked around. So much better! Would I do that again? I just wish I'd known what I knew this time around with my first and second!"

Mary Jane says, "After my fourth child (I have seven), I had no pain and was able to do anything. Walking and standing was the best way to speed things up."

The transition, or active, phase of labor begins at approximately 7 centimeters dilation and continues until full dilation (10 centimeters) and thinning of the cervix, or effacement (100 percent). This is the shortest phase, lasting 15 minutes to 1 hour, but the most intense. It ends at the second stage of labor.

In this phase, contractions become very intense and strong, and may even become erratic. With contractions coming every 1 to 2 minutes and lasting 60 to 90 seconds, you may not feel as if there is even a break between contractions. This is why it is important to rest in the early phases of labor to conserve energy.

Typically, if you have been able to stay relaxed, you will feel uncomfortable but in control. However, if you haven't been able to stay relaxed, you may feel as though you want to give up. You may be indecisive, restless, and irritable. The good news is that you may later experience natural amnesia and not remember this phase at all!

Hang in there! You're almost to the pushing stage. Remain focused and continue your relaxation, visualization, and breathing exercises. The more intense the contractions, the more you want to breathe deeply into the contraction. Picture your cervix opening like a blossom and relax your perineum. Picture your baby coming down to the light at the bottom of the birth canal. Try different positions. Sometimes rocking side-to-side is very comforting at this stage.

This is also the hardest part for your partner. No one wants to see his loved one in discomfort. But how your partner handles this phase will make a huge difference in your comfort level. Have your partner listen attentively to your needs and be sure he is prepared to make suggestions with various comfort measures because you may become very indecisive and the comfort measures that worked in early labor might not work now.

Women have a lot to say about the transition, or active, phase of labor. Roberta says, "With my third, I spent most of my hard labor time standing and leaning over the bed. I would bear down on it. Squatting seemed to feel pretty natural, too. I just let gravity do its work."

Karen says, "My first five labors progressed rapidly to classic transition. The contractions were intense; they started at my pelvis, moved up over my stomach and around like a tightening belt."

"I'm glad my husband made a cheat sheet for all the comfort measures I needed," says Maria. "Whenever he got flustered, he just reached into his pocket for ideas. I recommend all coaches bring a cheat sheet with them into the labor room."

Stage Two: Pushing

The pushing stage begins when the mother is fully dilated (10 centimeters) and effaced (100 percent) and ends with delivery of the infant. The duration can vary from 10 minutes to 3 or more hours. In this stage, contractions may have a period of ceasing. This is called the "rest and be thankful" stage. Then the contractions become more regular again, 2 to 5 minutes apart, and last 45 to 90 seconds. Many women report that these contractions are less painful and are usually accompanied by a strong urge to push.

Women usually get a second wind after laboring for many hours. You may find it easier to focus as you get to the last leg of your journey. Some women report a feeling of burning, stinging, or stretching as the baby comes down through the birth canal.

Question: One of my friends said that she never had the urge to push. I thought that every woman got it.

Answer: Every body is different. The majority of women do get an incredible, distinct, unavoidable, this-baby-is-coming urge to push. But there are some women who, for whatever reason, don't get this urge. Be sure to keep your body in an upright position (see illustration) so that gravity is helping to bring the baby down the birth canal. When it's time to push, you will know it!

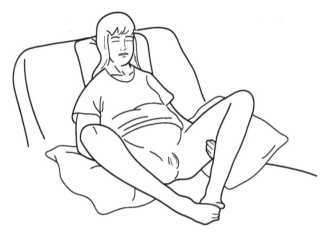

Go with your feelings. Gently push or breathe the baby out during a contraction. Between contractions, stay relaxed and focused. It usually relieves the contraction if you push during it. Try to find a position in which gravity can assist the baby's descent. Don't hold your breath for long periods. Let a small amount of air escape out of your mouth as you bear down, and take a new breath every 5 to 6 seconds. Keep your head in alignment with the spine and chin tucked in for optimal oxygen intake. If you want a chance to see your baby's head crown, mirrors usually are available.

If you are told that your baby is posterior, it is best to push while lying on your side. You will know if your baby is posterior if you felt labor in your back most of the time. This is commonly referred to as *back labor.* Alternate pushing 10 to 15 minutes on each side until the baby turns.

The labor coach is instrumental in helping the laboring mom get into positions that use gravity to help the baby's descent. Although it's very easy to get really excited and want to cheer her on like a fan at the Super Bowl, coaches should try to resist. Stay calm while encouraging her and remind her not to hold her breath. Climate control is still very important. Remember, this is the environment into which your baby is going to be born!

The pushing stage brings different recollections for different women. "When I was fully dilated," Judith says, "I didn't feel the urge to push and my contractions stopped, so my midwife let me rest until the contractions started again. I am so thankful she didn't try to rush things!"

Question: You keep mentioning that the coach should control the birthing environment. How much does this really matter?

Answer: Picture this—People are coming and going, talking loudly, cracking jokes, lights are on full-power, and a TV or radio is playing. Does this remind you of a party scene? Do you think you could relax during all this commotion? Most people couldn't. A quiet, calm atmosphere is much more conducive to relaxation. The lights should be dimmed, the door should be closed for privacy, visitors should be kept to a minimum (if any are present at all), the TV should be off, relaxation music may be played, and the temperature should be comfortable to Mom. Mom's job is to relax and work on birthing the baby. The coach's job is to support her and be her voice in relation to anything that affects the environment.

Roberta says, "I only got the urge to push when the baby had crowned. And he was coming whether I pushed or not! Once he hit the vaginal opening, there was a brief moment of burning and stinging. But that was it. Then he was in my arms!"

Stage Three: Afterbirth

This stage begins with the birth of the baby and ends with the delivery of the placenta and membranes. It usually lasts about 20 minutes, but most women are not even aware it is happening because they are holding their babies in their arms!

After the placenta is delivered, any stitching that needs to be done is performed. You will feel tired, but also euphoric. Birthing gives you a natural high. You may also feel cool and shaky. If the nurses do not offer you some warm blankets to ease the shakes, ask. Have skin-to-skin contact with your baby. Don't let the hospital staff wrap the baby all up in a blanket at this time. Your body heat will keep the baby warm.

If you're breast-feeding, try offering the infant the breast; she will be very receptive to it at this time and may even search it out if left on your abdomen. Relax, and know that you have done an awesome job. Welcome to motherhood!

The coach's job is to make sure Mom and baby are comfortable and are able to have time together immediately following birth, barring any medical problems. Keep the lights low. Remember, your baby just came from a nice dark, quiet place. Don't give him culture shock! When they take the baby to measure and bathe her, the coach should ask to go along, as long as Mom doesn't mind being left alone. If she does, the coach should stay with her. Report back to Mom with the stats, and let her know that the baby is doing fine. As soon as the staff is done doing what they need to, make sure the baby gets right back to Mom.

chapter 11

Adjusting During the Early Weeks After Delivery

Getting used to a new baby can be stressful in the early days after delivery, especially if you try to do everything. A baby can be very demanding on your time as well as your patience.

Remember that you are recovering from the childbirth experience, so listen to your body and try to do only what you comfortably can. There is nothing wrong with asking supportive friends and relatives to help you by cleaning the house, doing the laundry, or shopping for food. Save your energy for you and your baby.

Newborns are unpredictable, so it may be difficult for you to get enough sleep. Even if you are able to get enough total hours of sleep, you may not feel completely rested because your sleep cycles will be frequently interrupted. Try to nap during the day when the baby is napping and ask your partner to wake up during one of the night feedings. If you are breast-feeding, you can pump and store extra milk in the refrigerator, and once breast-feeding is well-established, you can ask your partner or others to give the baby a relief bottle at least once during the day or night.

Staying Well Nourished

A well-balanced diet is also important in making a healthful adjustment to the postpartum period. Many women want to lose the weight they've gained as quickly as possible. However, dieting can be dangerous while your body is recovering from pregnancy and childbirth. Instead, plan to eat nutritiously. Table 11.1 shows a sample food plan for new mothers.

Foods containing refined white flour and sugar or saturated fats should be used sparingly. Moderation is suggested for foods high in sodium, especially ketchup, soy sauce, bouillon, sauerkraut, and pickles. Read labels carefully.

Alcoholic beverages may be consumed in moderation, though you should avoid alcohol if breast-feeding. Limit caffeinated and carbonated beverages to two a day.

Question: Will breast-feeding help me lose weight faster?

Answer: There is a myth that breast-feeding will help you lose weight quickly. The reality is that your body will hold on to excess weight until the baby is about 6 months old, a time when the baby is typically introduced to solid food. This is the body's way of protecting the newborn from malnutrition. Plan to wear your maternity clothes home from the hospital or clothes with elastic waists for comfort.

TABLE 11.1 Meal Plan for Postpartum Women

| | | SERVINGS/DAY | |
Food	Serving size	Postpartum women	Lactating women
Whole grains	1 slice whole-grain bread 1/2 whole-grain bagel 1 ounce whole-grain cereal 1/2 cup brown rice or whole-grain pasta	6	9
Low-fat dairy	8 ounces skim milk 1.5 ounces natural cheese 2 ounces processed cheese 1 cup yogurt 1/2 cup ice cream	2	3
Fish, poultry, lean meat, eggs	3 to 4 ounces fish, poultry, lean meat 1 large egg 2 medium eggs	2	2
Nuts, legumes	1/4 cup nuts 1/2 cup dried beans or peas 2 tablespoons peanut butter	1	2
Vegetables	1 cup raw salad 1/2 cup vegetables, cooked or chopped 1/4 cup vegetable juice	At least 4	At least 4
Fruit*	1 medium piece of fruit 1/2 cup dried or cooked fruit 3/4 cup fruit juice	2	3
Plant oils	2 teaspoons	2	2

* Fresh fruit high in vitamin C is preferred.

If you eat healthfully and exercise moderately, eventually the excess weight will take care of itself. Try not to push it too fast. Hunger and fatigue can impede your recovery postpartum and can make you feel irritable and depressed.

In some cases, women feel blue or downright depressed after having a baby. This is often from the hormonal changes that occur after delivery. With proper diet, exercise, sleep, and adequate support from family and friends, you should be able to adjust in the most positive way possible. If you find, however, that you still feel sad after a couple of weeks, talk to your health care provider about various medications available to help elevate your mood after you have a baby.

Proper Body Mechanics for the New Mom

Taking care of a new baby can cause havoc on your lower back. All day long, you lean over a changing table, push a stroller, get the baby in and out of the car seat, and still try to complete your usual household chores. You will also find that because you are so focused on your newborn, you tend to be unaware of what is happening in your body most of the time. However, your body has a way of communicating with you when you are not paying attention—pain!

Don't wait for pain to motivate you to practice good body mechanics. Here are suggestions for preventing back problems after delivery:

Start with holding your baby. The best way to hold a newborn is in the center and close to your body (figure 11.1). Never put the baby on your hips, because it will create muscle imbalance and eventually lower back problems. Infant carriers and slings are also a great way to protect your back as well as free your arms to do other things.

When you purchase a stroller, be sure that you can comfortably walk with your elbows at a right angle (90 degrees) and in good posture (figure 11.2). You can also practice belly breathing and Kegel exercises as you walk.

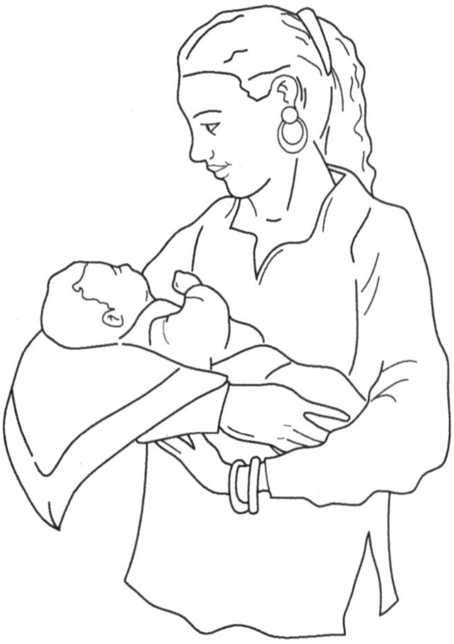

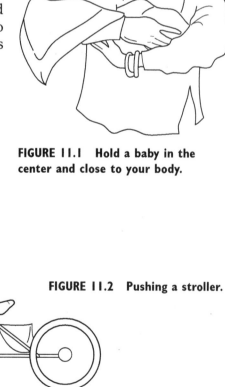

FIGURE 11.1   Hold a baby in the center and close to your body.

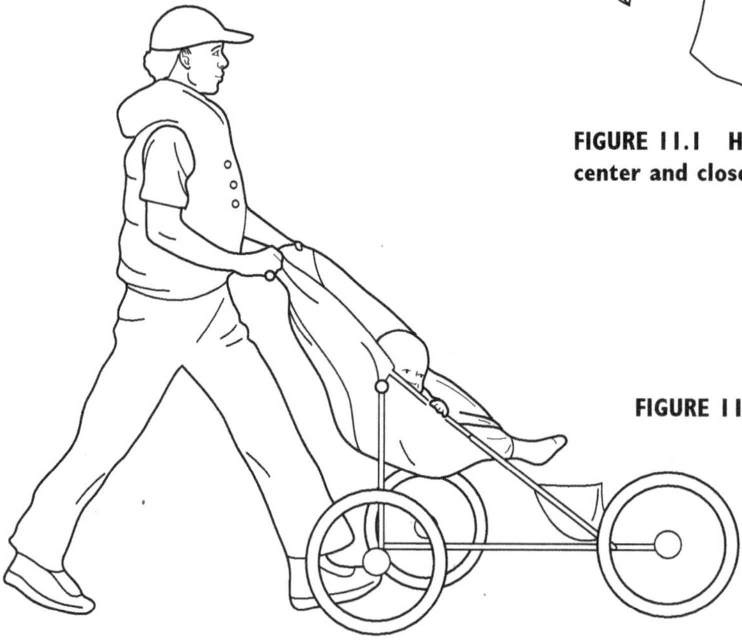

FIGURE 11.2   Pushing a stroller.

Avoid trying to put the baby into the car seat while you are outside the car. Hold your baby and get into the side of the car opposite the car seat. Once in the car and sitting on the seat, turn your whole body toward the car seat and then position baby safely. When it is time to get the baby out of the car seat, sit on the opposite side next to the car seat, remove the baby, and then carefully get out of the car.

Exercising After Delivery

The first few weeks after childbirth can be a hectic time for the new mother. Taking a shower may seem a big accomplishment! Although you might feel pressured for time, it is important to resume exercise as soon as you have permission from your health care provider. Typically providers recommend waiting until vaginal bleeding stops to resume a regular exercise regimen. Exercise will help you recover postpartum, return to prepregnancy proportions, and increase your energy. It took you 9 months to grow a baby, and it may take you up to 9 months to return to your prepregnancy shape. Be sensible, and take it slowly.

As soon as you can, start practicing Kegel exercises. Take a deep breath, and as you exhale, imagine pulling your vaginal opening up toward the inside of your belly button. Relax as you inhale and repeat the exercise 20 times, twice a day.

Practice the belly breathing exercise. Inhale while expanding your belly. As you exhale, pull your belly button toward your spine. Repeat this exercise 20 times, twice a day.

Drink lots of water before, during, and after exercise. Lactating moms should drink at least 8 ounces of water both before and after exercise. The best way to assess adequate hydration is to look at the color of your urine. Your urine should be a clear, pale yellow. If the urine appears darker, then you need to drink more water. Be sure to eat at regular intervals and include healthful snacks as well. A lactating mom should eat a piece of fruit, half a sandwich, or a salad after nursing and then after exercise.

Wear a supportive bra during exercise. If you need more support, try wearing two bras. Nurse before exercise for comfort. Studies show that moderate exercise does not affect your milk supply provided you drink lots of water. You may also want to wash your nipples after exercising and before nursing because babies tend to dislike the taste of sweat.

Get into a routine. Start by walking your baby for 15 minutes twice a day. Gradually increase your time as tolerated. Eventually, try to walk at least 30 minutes once a day or take two 20-minute walks on most days of the week.

The exercise session should feel good and enhance your feelings of well-being. Avoid exercising to fatigue. Start out slowly and plan to rest when the baby is sleeping at least once a day. There should be no pain or heavy bleeding associated with the exercise session. In fact, if you do experience heavy bleeding, stop exercising and see your health care provider. Sometimes, fragments of placenta tissue are left in the uterus. When this happens, heavy bleeding occurs periodically and the tissue needs to be removed as soon as possible. Doing too much, too soon, may also cause the site where the placenta was in the uterus to start to bleed again. Do not exercise if you experience heavy vaginal bleeding, pain, breast infection, or abscess.

For lactating moms, infant weight gain should be normal. If there is a problem, decrease exercise intensity and consult your health care provider. You may need to increase caloric intake to offset calories burned by exercise.

Getting to Know Your Newborn

The first month postpartum is a great time to get to know your baby. Even though you carried this child for 9 months or more, you may find that you look at your baby and wonder, *Who is this stranger?*

Now is a good time to really sharpen your listening skills. Babies communicate both verbally and nonverbally. If you *really* listen, you will notice subtle differences in the baby's cries, changes in expressions, as well as variations in body language. All of these cues are ways your baby communicates with you.

Newborn Reflexes

In addition to listening to your baby, you can also elicit certain newborn reflexes that tend to go unnoticed because many of them disappear about 4 to 6 months after birth. This is a way to learn about your baby as well as develop playing time. Often men become frustrated with infants because they are unable to verbalize their needs or play games. Now you both can have fun with your baby.

After your baby is fed, dry, and well-rested, spend some time with the baby's father and see if you can identify the reflexes described. Also, if you have any difficulty eliciting any of these reflexes, ask your baby's health care provider to demonstrate when you go for well-baby check-ups.

To elicit the palmer grasp, place your finger in the palm of baby's hand. Your infant's fingers curl around your fingers. Parents enjoy playing with this reflex. The palmer grasp disappears at 5 to 6 months of age.

The plantar grasp is a similar reflex for the feet. Elicit the response by placing your finger at the base of baby's toes. Baby's toes will curl downward. This reflex disappears at around 9 to 12 months.

For the Moro reflex, hold the baby in a semi-sitting position with your hands securely behind the back of the baby's head and shoulders. Allow the baby's head and trunk to slowly fall backward to an angle of 30 degrees.

Both of the baby's arms will extend outward. The fingers will fan out to form a C shape with the thumb and forefinger, then the arms will come together in an embracing motion. Report any asymmetrical response to your baby's health care provider because it may be a sign of injury to an arm or clavicle. The reflex disappears after 2 months.

The startle reflex can be elicited by loud hand clapping. The baby's arms will stretch with flexion of the elbows while the hands stay clenched. This response is easier to elicit in preterm babies. The reflex disappears at 4 months.

To elicit the gallant response, sometimes referred to as the swimming reflex, put your baby on his or her tummy. Stroke along the baby's spine on one side and then the other, alternating sides. The baby's torso will flex and his or her pelvis will swing toward the stimulated side. The reflex disappears around the fourth week.

Babies demonstrate a stepping or walking reflex even as newborns. To elicit the response, hold the baby vertically, allowing one foot to touch the surface. The baby will simulate walking, alternating flexion and extension of the feet. Full-term babies will step on the soles, while preterm babies will walk on their toes. The reflex lasts until about 2 months of age.

Stimulate the baby's foot to elicit Babinski's sign. On the sole of the baby's foot, begin touching the heel with one finger. Stroke upward on the outer side of the foot, then across the ball of the foot. The baby's big toe will flex while the other toes hyperextend. Absence of this sign should be reported to your baby's health care provider. The reflex disappears after 1 year.

Newborn Schedules

Many new parents try to make their babies fit into their schedules rather than take the baby's mood into consideration. Doing this with your baby might prove to be a disaster. Noticing your baby's states of consciousness will help you better learn why your infant might react to situations at different times and help you to plan activities around baby's ability to handle certain situations.

Throughout the day, babies go through six states of consciousness that affect their bodies, breathing, and levels of response. The more you understand your baby's states of consciousness, the easier it will be to avoid uncomfortable situations. As an example, if you notice that your baby is in the active alert stage while you are having company, it might be best not to have people pick the baby up at this time. Otherwise, you will probably have a crying baby on your hands. Table 11.2 lists the states of consciousness as well as what to expect.

One of the hardest things about having a new baby is when your baby cries and you just don't know what to do. All babies cry 1 to 2 hours each day. It's the only way they can communicate their needs and get rid of frustration. However, some babies cry more than others.

TABLE 11.2 States of Consciousness

State	Body activity	Eye movement	Facial movement	Breathing pattern	Level of response
Deep sleep	Nearly still except for an occasional twitch	None	Without facial expression	Smooth and regular	Threshold to stimuli very high; hard to arouse
Light sleep	Some body movement	Rapid eye movements (REM)	May smile and make brief fussy or crying sounds	Irregular	More responsive to internal and external stimuli
Drowsy	Activity level is variable	Eyes open and close occasionally; dull, glazed appearance; heavy lidded	May have some facial movements	Irregular	Delayed reaction to sensory stimuli; state may change after baby is stimulated
Quiet alert	Minimal	Brightening and widening of eyes	Face looks bright and sparkling	Regular	Optimum state of arousal; infant attentive to the environment
Active alert	Much body activity; periods of fussiness	Eyes open with less brightness	Much facial movement	Irregular	Sensitive to disturbing stimuli such as hunger, fatigue, noise, and excessive handling
Crying	Increased motor activity with skin color change	Eyes either tightly closed or open	Grimaces	More irregular	Extreme response to unpleasant internal or external stimuli

If your baby cries more than 4 hours a day for no apparent reason, chances are he or she is sensitive. Pediatricians and parents alike often refer to these babies as having *colic,* but this term has a negative connotation and implies that the baby is being bad.

There is nothing either good or bad, but thinking makes it so.

Shakespeare, Hamlet act II, scene II

About 1 out of 3 infants is a sensitive baby. Usually, infants grow out of this sensitivity around 3 months of age. Typically, the baby will have crying bouts that last 4 to 5 minutes, then will settle down and start to cry again. Nothing seems to soothe the infant. This can be quite frustrating to the new parents. Crying seems to be more common in the afternoon and evening when the baby is tired. However, no one really knows the exact cause.

Researchers do know that first-born children tend to be more sensitive in the first couple of months than second or third babies. There may also be a relationship between excessive crying and a difficult birth. Stress and isolation have also been found to play a role. Other theories include trapped air in the stomach and intestines, cow's milk formula, and an immature neurological system.

Observe your baby and notice when and where he or she cries for no apparent reason. Be compassionate rather than irritated. Try to imagine what it feels like to be in discomfort and not be able to communicate your feelings.

Here are some strategies to help soothe your baby. Try each one separately for 4 to 5 days to see if any work for your baby.

- If using a cow's milk based formula, switch to a soy-based formula for a few days.
- If breast-feeding, stay away from cow's milk products including cheese, ice cream, and yogurt, but remember to take a calcium supplement.
- If bottle feeding, try to reduce the amount of air your baby is swallowing during mealtimes by making sure that the nipple holes in the bottle are not too big.
- Burp the baby frequently while feeding.
- Try to reduce distractions during feeding times.
- Stay calm. Your baby can sense when you are stressed and may act out of your frustration. Use your relaxation breathing techniques as you hold the baby close to your chest.
- Limit the amount of stimulus your baby is exposed to.
- Take your baby for a ride in the car or sit the car seat on top of the dryer. Vibrations often help soothe babies. Do not leave the baby unattended.
- Move the baby's legs in toward the belly and then straighten them outward. This may help relieve gas (figure 11.3).
- Keep the baby away from cigarette smoke or other toxic odors.
- Try to swaddle or massage your baby.

Some pediatric health care providers recommend certain medicines or herbs to give your baby relief from any abdominal discomfort that may be causing excessive crying. Simethicone drops seem to help get rid of intestinal gas and have no side effects. Check with your provider before giving your baby any over-the-counter remedies.

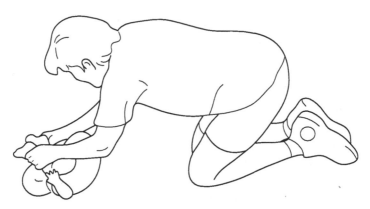

FIGURE 11.3   Moving a baby's legs toward the belly and then straightening them may help relieve gas.

Infant Massage

One of the earliest senses your baby develops is the sense of touch. Research has shown that touch is as important to infant survival as eating and sleeping. Skin stimulation, in fact, has been proven to be essential for adequate organ and psychological development for both animals and humans.

Massage also improves circulation, stimulates the digestive system, enhances neurological development, helps muscle tone, and has a calming effect on the baby. Most important, it is an enjoyable way for you and other members of you family to interact with your baby in positive ways.

Question: I want to massage my baby, but every time I try, she cries and seems irritable. What do you recommend?

Answer: Not all infants enjoy massage at first. If your baby gets cranky or looks away, stop and try another time. Even a baby who enjoys massages may not enjoy it every time. Become aware of those times when your baby just needs some quiet time. The best time to massage your baby is when he or she is in the quiet, alert state of consciousness.

Pay attention to the amount of pressure you use. Infant massage is a surface massage, rather than a deep massage. Every stroke should be gentle and slow. Often you will use one finger or part of your hand rather than your whole hand. At first, use downward strokes, which are more calming. Upward strokes are more stimulating.

Babies are usually more sensitive on their chests and faces. Avoid these areas if massaging them seems to irritate your baby.

Use vegetable oil instead of lotion because babies usually put their hands in their mouths while getting massaged. Always warm the oil in your hands before rubbing it on the baby. Trim your nails and remove any jewelry on your wrists and hands. Keep eye contact and softly speak or sing to your baby. Try to do the massage in the same order so baby can get used to a routine.

Avoid giving a massage to your baby at least 48 hours after getting a shot, while baby is sick, or within an hour and a half after feeding. Avoid the soft spots on your baby's head.

Pick a time when your baby is most relaxed, either in the morning or after an evening bath. Use a baby blanket to cover the parts of the baby not being massaged. This provides warmth and comfort.

Choose a place that is warm, quiet, and comfortable for both you and your baby. Place your baby on a firm surface, either the floor or changing table. Keep a diaper on your baby or underneath the baby's bottom. Turn on the answering machine or take the phone off of the hook. Be sure pets are also out of the room, especially if you are massaging your baby on the floor.

Before massaging your baby, say your baby's name and ask permission to massage. Plan to spend 10 to 30 minutes massaging your baby.

Start with the baby's legs and feet. With the baby lying on her back, loosely wrap both of your hands around one leg. With slight pressure, make long, sweeping motions from the baby's hip to the foot. Alternate with your right and left hands. Move your thumbs up and down the baby's foot, pressing thumb over thumb, gently massaging the bottom of the foot. Knead each toe by gently squeezing and pulling each one. This is a good time to sing "This Little Piggy". Roll one leg between both of your hands (like playing with modeling clay). Make small circles around the ankles. Pat the leg and lightly stroke to finish. Repeat everything on the other leg.

Well, the first days are the hardest days, don't you worry anymore.

Jerry Garcia

Move to the baby's arms and hands. Hold one of the baby's arms and gently pat to relax. With the tips of your fingers, make small circles in the armpit. As with the legs, gently stroke the arms toward the fingers using the hand-over-hand technique. Open the palm and massage the hand. Knead every finger. This is a good time to sing nursery rhymes that use the fingers. Roll the arm between both of your hands, working down the arm. End by gently stroking the arm and repeat the sequence on the other arm.

Massage the baby's tummy. With the outside of your right hand, stroke downward on the baby's tummy. Keep the hand slightly cupped, almost in a scooping motion. Then do the same with the left hand. Use the hand-over-hand technique. Put both of your thumbs at the midline of the baby's abdomen and gently press outward below and above the belly button. Rotate your hands clockwise, making circular motions on the abdomen.

Move to the baby's chest. With your fingertips, start at the center of the chest and circle outward so your hands are going in opposite directions. Draw an imaginary heart on the baby's chest. Stroke from the opposite shoulder to the opposite hip, alternating sides.

Turn the baby onto her stomach either on the floor, changing table, or across your lap to massage her back. Place your hands on each side of the baby's spine and gently stroke up and down the spine in sweeping motions. Do not put any pressure directly over the spine. Stroke sideways across the width of the back, alternating hands and traveling up and down the back. Make small circles upward along the sides of the spine and then continue the circling motion over the shoulders. Make small circles downward along the sides of the spine and then continue the motion around the buttocks. On both sides of the spine, lightly stroke from the shoulders down to the heels and back up again. End by patting and lightly stroking the back.

If you feel you need some formal training, look in your area for infant massage classes or watch one of the many videos available. As long as you follow the guidelines and massage with an intention of love, you really can't do anything wrong. And who knows, maybe some day your grown-up baby will give you a massage.

Fitness for
the New Mom

Babies do not come with instructions. Much of parenting involves trial and error. To have a positive parenting experience, you need to learn about your baby inside and out.

When your baby was born, you carefully examined him physically to be sure there were 10 fingers and 10 toes. Now you need to learn about what is happening on the inside. How does your baby react to certain situations? What are your baby's biological rhythms? What are your baby's likes and dislikes?

Each child is unique. Every baby is born with innate characteristics that, for the most part, determine how she responds to various environmental stimuli. These characteristics are called *temperament*. After about 2 months, you may start to notice some consistencies in your baby's behavior. Observe your baby over the next couple of weeks and note his behavior in the following areas:

- Regularity—predictability of biological functioning, such as feeding, sleeping, and waste elimination
- Activity level—motor activity and the proportion of active and inactive periods
- Sensory threshold—level of stimulation needed to evoke a response
- Adaptability—response to change in daily routines or new experiences
- Mood—your baby's overall attitude (happy, neutral, fussy, crying)
- Distractibility—effectiveness of outside stimuli on changing behavior
- Attention span—duration an activity is pursued without interruption

After observing your baby's behavior, you may be better able to anticipate needs. Remember, though, as baby grows and changes, parents need to adapt parenting to meet these needs. Becoming familiar with your baby's pattern of behavior will make the times of change a lot easier.

Sexual Health After Delivery

Adjusting to the new roles of parenthood can be an exciting, yet extremely challenging part of life. Many aspects of daily living are altered and you need to adapt to new demands and growing responsibilities.

Amidst all of these changes, sexual concerns are frequently overlooked. It is important, though, that you and your partner resume sexual relations in the most satisfying ways possible. Just as it takes time for you to feel comfortable about baby care, it may take a while before lovemaking returns to normal.

Before resuming sex, check with your health care provider to be sure that you are physically healthy. Also, you need to decide on an appropriate birth-control method if you choose not to become pregnant again right away. Some women believe that breast-feeding inhibits ovulation. In some cases it does, but although you do not have a menstrual period while you are breastfeeding, you may still be ovulating. It is always a good idea to talk to your health care provider about birth control before leaving the hospital. However, many providers wait until the first post-partum visit.

After delivering a baby, you may find that you have very little interest in sex. Biological changes as well as new demands on time and energy can sap physical desire. Here are the five most common reasons new moms tend to experience a drop in sexual desire:

1. After delivery, the new mom experiences a drop in hormones. Couples may experience frustration if there are changes in the woman's physiologic response to sexual stimulation. The decrease in sexual desire caused by the drop in hormones may inhibit sexual responses for 2 to 3 months after delivery. In addition, the new mom's body image may be temporarily altered. Exercise and eating nutritiously will help provide additional energy and a greater sense of well-being.

2. Fatigue is a common experience after delivering a baby. Excessive fatigue may decrease normal sexual desire. At least once a day, try to sleep when your baby sleeps.

3. Many new moms experience a fear of pain. Depending on the type of delivery experienced, the new mom might have stitches that need to heal. Some women also have breast tenderness whether they are breast-feeding or not. To prepare for intercourse, insert a clean finger into your vaginal opening and note whether you have any discomfort. You might also want to use a lubricant because a drop in estrogen levels may make you dry.

4. Stress is a natural part of being a new parent. When you are always thinking about meeting the baby's needs, it is hard to shift your focus on doing something just for yourself. If you find you are tense and unable to relax, ask your partner to give you a gentle massage while you practice some of the relaxation techniques you used in labor.

5. Finally, lack of opportunity may decrease the occurrence of sexual activity. There is no rule that sex has to be a nighttime event. Try having sex during the day whenever you get the chance. Be creative!

Discomfort during intercourse is common the first time after having baby, but do not despair. The breathing and relaxation exercises you practiced during pregnancy can also be useful during lovemaking.

If you are breastfeeding, you may also find that becoming excited causes milk to spurt from your nipples. Some couples find this amusing. If it bothers you, try to wear a nursing bra with nursing pads during sexual intercourse. It is also common for a woman to become sexually aroused when breastfeeding because of the hormone released during nursing. Remember, these are all normal responses.

Relationship issues sometimes surface after the birth of a baby. Hopefully, you have developed good communication skills with your partner. Even if you are not interested in sex initially, your partner is probably anxious to get things back to normal.

People have a tendency to assume their partner can read their minds. Don't fall into this trap! Chances are, if you don't tell your partner what you need and want, he will not know how to please you. Be compassionate to your partner's needs, just as you want him to be compassionate to your needs. If you really are not physically or emotionally prepared to resume intercourse, discuss this with your partner. There are many other ways to be intimate.

Even when you are tired from taking care of the baby 24/7, being close to another adult helps refill your energy tank. Also if you communicate with your partner, he might be able to help you find ways to decrease your stress.

Make a plan to go on a date with your partner—just the two of you—by 2 months after you deliver. Ask a relative or friend to stay with the baby, even for just an hour or so, so you both can get reacquainted. Go to dinner or a movie or exercise together. Keep the lines of communication going. But most of all, enjoy the excitement of rediscovering each other.

Exercising After the First Month Postpartum

Exercise during the first couple of months after delivery will help you feel more emotionally stable and reduce hot flashes and night sweats that frequently occur until your ovarian function returns to normal. It will also help get you back to exercising on a regular basis. Studies show that the longer the new mother puts off exercising, the less likely she will exercise at all.

Most women do not want to leave their babies during this honeymoon phase. For that reason, exercising with your baby is an ideal solution. Weight-bearing exercise such as walking is best because it stimulates bone density, which has been shown to decrease about 5 percent over the initial 3 months after delivery from a drop in hormone levels.

Exercise classes designed especially for moms and babies are an excellent way to get the needed exercise and, just as important, network with other new moms. Sometimes finding time to attend a class is difficult, but it is worth the effort. The key is to plan ahead and get everything ready the night before. Preparing the diaper bag ahead of time, including a water bottle for yourself, will help reduce the mad rush out the door. It also becomes a motivator for actually going to the class. After all, if everything is ready, you have no excuses.

Walking is a perfect exercise for the new mom, and getting out in the fresh air also benefits baby. You can either walk with your baby in a front infant carrier or use a stroller. If you choose to use a stroller, be sure that the handles are tall enough to allow your elbows to be bent at a 90-degree angle. As with any exercise, be sure to stay in good posture and stretch after each walk to keep your muscles healthy.

Another good weight-bearing exercise is dancing with your baby. Not only will you feel better, the movement and music may stimulate infant development and, if nothing else, put the baby to sleep. Just turn on the music, put your baby in a front infant carrier for safety, and have a ball! Incorporate stretching into your dance routine as well.

Shaping up after delivery is an ongoing process. It usually takes a new mom 6 months to a year to return to prepregnancy proportions. You will reap many benefits by starting to exercise early in the postpartum phase and continuing on a regular basis. Eventually, regular, sustained exercise will help you return to your prepregnancy weight, improve abdominal muscle tone, and enhance your overall body image.

Question: What works best for losing weight—dieting or exercise?

Answer: The combination of exercise and diet is best. Researchers have found that short-term weight loss (about 1 kilogram, or 2 pounds, a week) through a combination of diet and exercise appears to be the best way to lose weight after delivery. Weight loss achieved primarily through dieting without exercise reduces maternal lean body mass, lowering metabolism and making it even harder to shed those unwanted pounds. The slower you lose the weight, the more chance you have for keeping it off for good!

Continue to perform at least 20 Kegel exercises at least twice a day every day. Try to walk 20 to 30 minutes a day and gradually work up to 45 minutes at a good pace at which you can talk, but you can't sing. You might want to split your aerobic workouts by walking your baby twice a day for 15 to 20 minutes each time.

In addition, work on strengthening your core muscles because abdominal muscles were stretched and chances are they need to be toned. Here are some key exercises to practice along with instructions for breathing while you practice core exercises. The core exercises are designed to both strengthen and stretch the muscles of the core. The core exercises are listed in the order of intensity. Start with the first exercise and slowly progress according to your individual comfort and tolerance level.

Breathing Basics

With all exercises, the breathing pattern needs to be well established. Also be aware of stabilizing the spine before movement actually takes place. Inhale and exhale through the nose, or inhale through the nose and exhale through pursed lips. Try to breathe as deeply as possible, expanding the rib cage as you inhale and pressing the abdominal wall toward the spine as you exhale. Practice holding the abdominal muscles toward the spine and breathing into the sides and back of your torso.

When breathing consciously, only the muscles of the torso are working. Think about relaxing the muscles in the shoulders, neck, arms, and legs. Stay focused on the breath during all exercises. Through awareness of the breath, the mind–body connection is strengthened. When in doubt, just breathe!

Question: I can't breathe through my nose because of sinus problems. What do you recommend?

Answer: The ideal is to breathe in and out through your nose. However, if breathing through your nose is difficult, just breathe in a way that is most comfortable for you.

Lying Pelvic Tilt

Lie on your back with the knees bent and the feet flat on the floor. Keep the hands relaxed at your sides. As you exhale, pull your belly toward your spine, tilting your pelvis forward (figure 12.1). As you inhale, release. In this position, feel the weight of your sacrum releasing to the floor. Repeat the exercise 8 to 10 times.

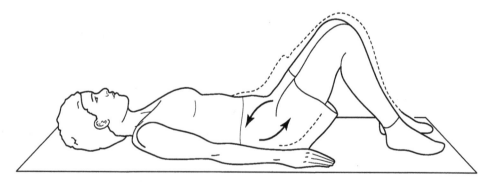

FIGURE 12.1   Lying pelvic tilt.

Heel Slides

Lie on your back with the knees bent and the feet flat on the floor. As you inhale, slide your right foot forward until your leg is straight (figure 12.2). Keep your lower back pressed to the floor. Exhale and bring your leg back in. Repeat the exercise on the other side. Alternate sides 5 to 10 times.

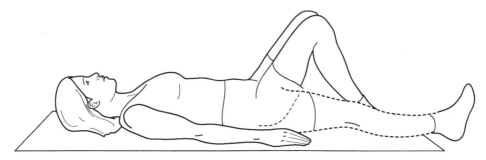

FIGURE 12.2   Heel slide.

Single-Foot Touch

Lie on your back with your knees bent at a 90-degree angle over your hips. As you inhale, place your right foot on the floor while keeping your lower back pressed into the floor (figure 12.3). As you exhale, bring your foot back up. Repeat the exercise on the other side. Alternate sides 5 to 10 times.

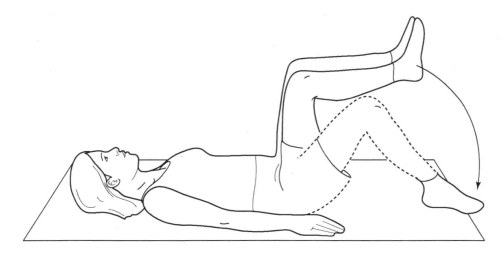

FIGURE 12.3   Single-foot touch.

Double-Foot Touch

Start in the same position as the single-foot touch. Inhale and place both feet on the floor while keeping your lower back on the floor (figure 12.4). As you exhale, bring both legs back up. Repeat the exercise 5 to 10 times.

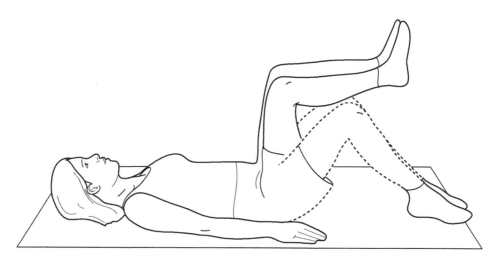

FIGURE 12.4   Double-foot touch.

Basic Bridge

Lie on your back with the knees bent and both feet flat on the floor. As you exhale, tilt the hips forward and lift up (figure 12.5). Hold this position for 2 to 3 breath cycles. As you exhale, slowly lower your hips, feeling each vertebra one at a time. Repeat the exercise 5 to 10 times.

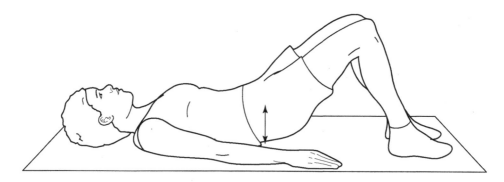

FIGURE 12.5   Basic bridge.

Progressive Bridge

Start from a basic bridge position. As you exhale, squeeze buttocks muscles and lift your hips, waist, and rib cage (figure 12.6). Hold this position for 2 to 3 breath cycles and then lower slowly, releasing the rib cage, waist, and hips back to the floor, feeling each vertebra one at a time. Repeat the exercise 5 to 10 times.

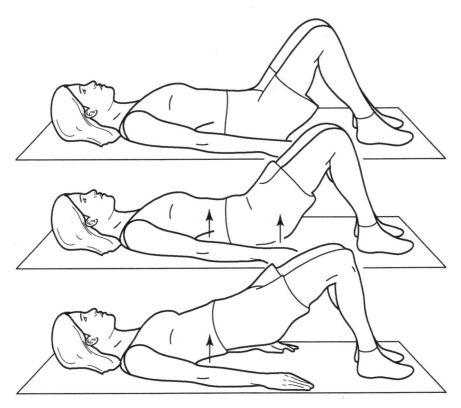

FIGURE 12.6 Progressive bridge.

Alternating Bridge

Start from a basic bridge position. Slowly roll up to a progressive bridge. As you inhale, bring your right hip to the floor. As you exhale, lift your right hip back up. Repeat the exercise on the other side. Alternate sides 5 to 10 times.

Hundreds

Start on your back with the knees bent. As you contract your abdominal muscles, lift your head to look at your belly button. Slide your scapula down your back to stabilize the shoulders. Stretch the arms along the sides of the torso with the palms facing down about 6 inches off the floor (figure 12.7). Inhale for 5 counts while pulsing the arms downward (like slapping the air above the floor) and then exhale for 5 counts as you continue to pulse the arms. Repeat the movement for 10 breath cycles, a total of 100 counts.

To increase the intensity of the exercise, lift the feet off the floor so the heels are in line with the knees and the calves are parallel to the floor. To further increase the intensity, straighten the legs up to the ceiling or lower slightly toward the floor as long as you can keep the lower back pressed to the floor.

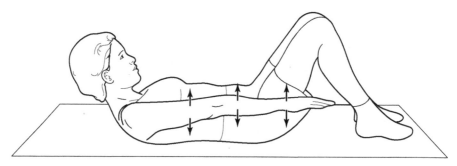

FIGURE 12.7 Hundreds.

After finishing hundreds, relax with this exercise: Lie on your back with the knees bent in toward the torso and the feet off the floor. Wrap your arms around your knees or behind your thighs and gently rock from side to side (figure 12.8).

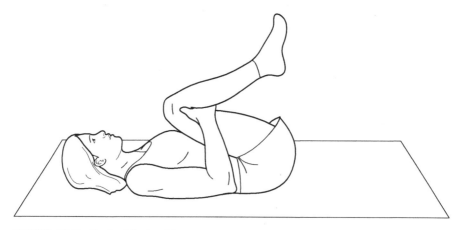

FIGURE 12.8 Rock side to side.

Roll-Ups

Lie on your back. Press your belly button toward the spine so that the lower back is pressing toward the floor. Bend the legs at the knees or stretch them out on the floor with the feet flexed. As you inhale, raise your arms toward the ceiling and start to roll up to a sitting position. Face the palms inward. As you exhale, round the back into a C curve, reaching the arms toward the feet (figure 12.9). As you inhale, straighten the spine. Exhale, lightly pointing the toes and slowly rolling back down. Repeat the exercise for a total of 5 to 8 times.

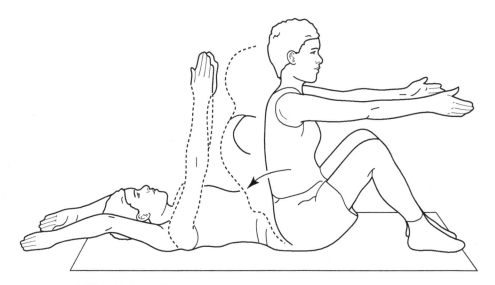

FIGURE 12.9   Roll-ups.

When rolling up and rolling down, start each movement with a posterior pelvic tilt to decrease stress on the lower back. To decrease the intensity, bend the knees while rolling up and then straighten for the remainder of the exercise.

If you are not able to roll up with the legs bent or straight, sit straight up with the knees bent, feet the flat on the floor, and hands resting on your knees. On the exhalation, round the back. On the inhalation, straighten up. Repeat this exercise 5 to 8 times.

Rolling

Sit tall with the knees bent and the arms holding the legs, either below the knees or behind the thighs. Lean back slightly and balance with the feet off the floor. Initiate the roll by exhaling and pulling the abdominal muscles toward the spine. This increases the flexion of the lumbar spine (lower back). Roll backward no further than the thoracic spine (middle back) (figure 12.10). As you inhale, roll back to the starting position and straighten your spine while balancing on the coccyx area (base of your spine). Roll for about 8 to 10 repetitions. To increase the intensity, keep the knees at a 90-degree angle with the calves parallel to the floor.

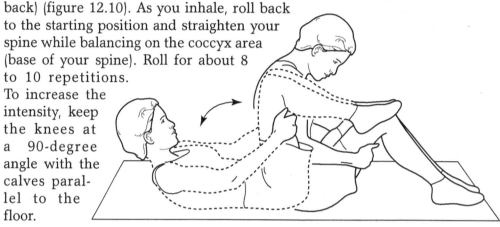

FIGURE 12.10   Rolling.

Single Leg Stretch

Lie on your back with the upper body lifted off the mat. Bend the knees at a 90-degree angle with the hands resting against the outside of the legs. Exhale and extend the right leg forward about a foot off the floor while moving the left hand to the left ankle and right hand to the left knee, pulling the left knee towards chest (figure 12.11). Inhale and switch legs and hands. Exhale and extend the left leg and move the hands to the right leg and pull the right knee towards chest. Alternate sides for 8 to 10 repetitions. Bring both knees toward the chest and rest.

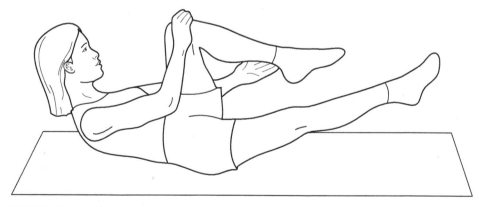

FIGURE 12.11   Single-leg stretch.

Oblique Strengtheners

Lie on the floor with the knees bent at a 90-degree angle. Place your hands behind your head with the fingertips lightly touching each side of the head and elbows out to the sides. Relax your shoulders away from your ears. As you exhale, extend one leg while rotating the torso toward the other leg, reaching the armpit to the opposite knee (figure 12.12). Keep the extended leg above the floor at a level that allows you to keep the lower back pressed to the floor. As you inhale, switch legs and turn the torso to the other side so the other armpit is reaching toward the opposite knee. Alternate sides for a total of 8 to 10 repetitions. To decrease the intensity, keep the knees bent with feet flat on the floor and alternate rotating the torso only.

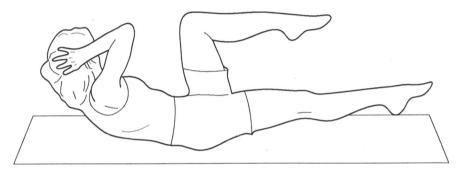

FIGURE 12.12   Oblique strengthener.

Single-Leg Kick

Lie on your stomach with the elbows under the shoulders. Prop your torso on your forearms with your chest lifted off the mat. Legs are extended with feet lightly pointed. Pull the belly button toward the spine to stabilize the back. As you exhale, bend one leg toward the buttock with two controlled pulses. On the first pulse, flex the foot (figure 12.13). On the second pulse, lightly point the toes. As you inhale, straighten the leg. Alternate legs for a total of 5 to 8 repetitions on each side. If you have lower back discomfort, try this modification: Instead of lifting the torso off the floor, rest your forehead on your hands and leave the chest on the floor.

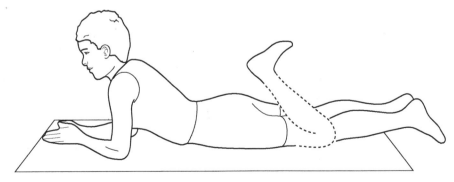

FIGURE 12.13   Single-leg kick.

Swimmer

Lie on your stomach with your arms stretched out in front of shoulders, your palms turned down, and the head and shoulders lifted off the floor. Press the shoulders away from your ears to stabilize the torso. Pull the abdomen in so your belly button is pressed toward your spine. As you inhale, raise the opposite arm and opposite leg off the floor (figure 12.14). Exhale and relax. Alternate sides for a total of 5 to 8 repetitions.

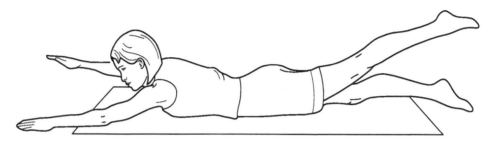

FIGURE 12.14   Swimmer.

Question: I am breast-feeding, and when I lie on my stomach, my breasts are uncomfortable. How can I exercise on my belly without being uncomfortable?

Answer: Before you are ready to exercise, breast-feed your baby. This will decrease the amount of milk in your breasts and will help make you more comfortable. You can also put a pillow under your chest.

Side Kicks

Lie on your right side with the right arm under your head and the left arm resting in front of your torso. Bring your legs together and slightly in front of the hips. Lift the top leg and move it forward and backward, keeping the foot flexed and torso stationary (figure 12.15). Repeat the exercise 6 times. Roll over and repeat the exercise on the other side.

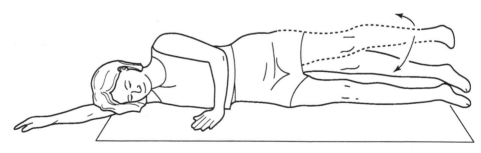

FIGURE 12.15   Side kicks.

Cool-Down

After performing core exercises, bring balance back into your body by performing the stretching exercises described in chapter 1. Specifically, perform the rounded cat stretch (page 6), quadriceps stretch (page 13), monkey stretch (page 14), shoulder stretch (page 15), standing torso stretch (page 15), and standing forward bend (page 17). If you are having any back discomfort, instead of the standing forward bend, do the wall-supported back stretch (page 16).

Exercising With Baby

Finding time to exercise after having a baby can be a challenge, especially for women who are breast-feeding. Many moms take walks with the baby in a stroller but rarely have an opportunity to strengthen and tone specific muscles affected by pregnancy.

Both mother and baby enjoy the interaction that exercising together brings. Exercising with your infant helps promote bonding, gives you a chance to shape up without needing a babysitter, and even stimulates infant development. Teach Dad these exercises, too—he may benefit from them as well!

Keep these tips in mind when planning to exercise with your baby:

- Only exercise with your baby if he or she seems to like participating. The best time is half an hour after eating, and when baby's diaper is clean.
- Hold the baby with both hands when he is sitting or lying on top of your thighs or torso.
- Avoid jerky or extremely bouncy movements.
- If the baby is unable to support her head (less than 6 months old), keep both hands behind her head when she is not resting on the floor.
- Talk to your baby and have fun!

Baby Sit-Ups

Sit up straight with the soles of your feet together, knees apart. Lay your baby on his back with his upper torso on your feet. Grab the baby's hands, supporting his head if necessary. Pull your belly toward your spine and round your back as you bring your baby toward your chest. Gently pull your baby to a sitting or standing position as you roll your spine down toward the floor (figure 12.16). Remember, the lower you go, the harder it is to come back up. Only go as far back as you comfortably can. Pull the abdominal muscles toward the spine. As you inhale, sit back up, slowly bringing the baby back toward your feet. Repeat the exercise 3 to 5 times.

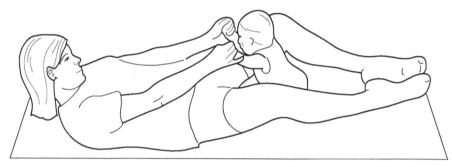

FIGURE 12.16   Baby sit-ups.

Baby Presses

Lie on your back with your knees bent. Hold your baby between your hands. Pull your abdomen toward your spine and press your lower back toward the floor. As you exhale, extend your arms while lifting the baby up (figure 12.17). As you inhale, bend your elbows and bring the baby back to your chest. Repeat the exercise 6 to 8 times.

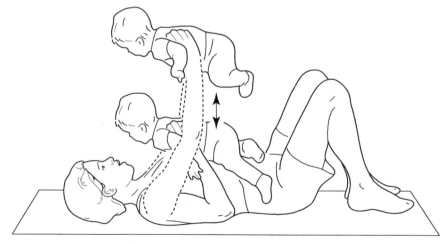

FIGURE 12.17   Baby presses.

Kiss the Baby

Get into a tabletop position with your back straight. Lay the baby below your chest. Keeping your hips over your knees, inhale while bending the elbows and bringing the chest toward the floor (figure 12.18). Kiss the baby. As you exhale, straighten your elbows and return to starting position. Repeat the exercise 6 to 8 times. If you find this exercise to be easy, perform a modified push-up with shoulders and hips in alignment and lifting your feet off the floor while keeping knees bent.

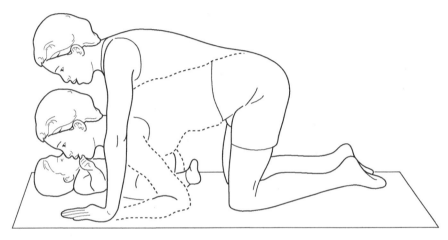

FIGURE 12.18   Kiss the baby.

Back Strengthener With Baby

Get into a tabletop position with the baby lying on a mat or blanket below you. Tighten your abdomen to stabilize the spine. Extend the opposite arm and leg and balance (figure 12.19). Keep the back toes touching the floor if balancing is difficult. Hold the position for 3 to 5 breaths. Repeat the exercise on the other side. Alternate sides twice.

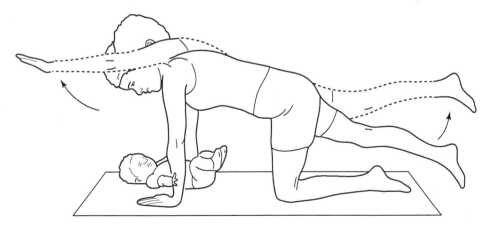

FIGURE 12.19   Back strengthener with baby.

Downward Facing Baby

From a tabletop position with the baby lying on a mat or blanket below you, straighten the legs and lift the buttocks toward the ceiling. Pull back in the hips, shifting your weight onto your heels (figure 12.20). Hold the position for 3 to 5 breaths. Bend the knees and rest.

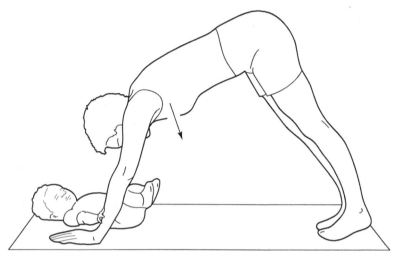

FIGURE 12.20   Downward facing baby.

Baby Bridges

Lie on your back with the baby sitting on your belly and resting against your thighs. Hold him with both hands to keep him from falling to one side. Exhale, squeeze your buttocks, and lift your hips off the floor (figure 12.21). Inhale and relax. Exhale and lift your hips and waist off the floor. Inhale and slowly roll down. Exhale and lift your hips, waist and, rib cage off the floor. Inhale and slowly roll down, feeling each vertebra, one at a time. Repeat the sequence one more time. In this position, you can also practice the alternating bridge exercise, described on page 191.

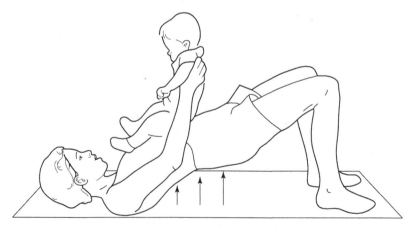

FIGURE 12.21   Baby bridges.

Lifetime Fitness for the Whole Family

With the birth of a baby come new beginnings. You will find yourself growing and learning along with your baby. Now that you are exercising regularly, try to incorporate exercise into family activities. Babies learn by modeling their parents. The more you practice a healthful lifestyle, the better the chance that your children will follow in your footsteps. Here are some tips for family fun and fitness:

- Plan family fitness time at least twice a week. Try to get on a regular schedule.
- Choose activities that allow everyone to participate.
- Follow good exercise principles, including warming up, cooling down, and stretching.
- Include other family members such as aunts, uncles, and cousins, if possible.
- Emphasize the importance of having fun. Avoid being competitive.
- Use physical activity, not food, as a reward.
- Select fitness-oriented gifts for birthdays and holidays.
- Keep fresh fruits and vegetables washed, cut up, and ready to eat for quick snacks.
- Always use the stairs going down and going up, if you and your family can tolerate it.
- Take a family fitness vacation such as skiing, canoeing, camping, or hiking.
- Dance with your family.
- Provide space in your yard for sports such as Frisbee, basketball, and football.

By encouraging your children to exercise regularly, you will help them avoid obesity in adulthood as well as all of the diseases that are associated with being overweight and out-of-shape such as diabetes, heart disease, various cancers, and joint problems.

You worked hard to have a healthy baby. Keep your momentum going by planning to have a healthy family!

bibliography

American Academy of Pediatrics and American College of Obstetricians and Gynecologists. 2002. *Guidelines for perinatal care* (fifth ed.). Elk Grove Village, Illinois: American Academy of Pediatrics. Washington, DC: American College of Obstetricians and Gynecologists.

American College of Obstetricians and Gynecologists. 2000. *Planning your pregnancy and birth* (third ed.). Washington, DC: American College of Obstetricians and Gynecologists.

Clapp, J.F., MD. 2002. *Exercising through your pregnancy.* Omaha, Nebraska: Addicus Books, Inc.

McClure, V.S. 2000. *Infant massage: A handbook for loving parents.* New York: Bantam Books.

Mittlemark, R.A., Wiswell, R.A., and Drinkwater, B.L. 1991. *Exercise in pregnancy* (second ed.). Baltimore: Williams & Wilkins.

Khalsa, Shakta Kaur. 2002. *Yoga for women.* New York: DK Publishing.

Mayo Clinic. 1994. *Mayo Clinic complete book of pregnancy and baby's first year.* New York: William Morrow and Company, Inc.

Mongan, M.F. 1998. *Hypnobirthing: A celebration of life.* Concord, New Hampshire: Rivertree.

MOTHERWELL *Yoga Video for Expectant Moms.* 2001. Boiling Springs, Pennsylvania: Classic Video Productions. To order, visit www.motherwellfitness.com or call 1-800-MOMWELL.

Zi, Nancy. 1997. *The Art of Breathing* (third ed.). Glendale, California: Vivi Co.

Web Site Resources

Agency for Healthcare Research and Quality	www.ahcpr.gov
American Academy of Pediatrics	www.aap.org
The American College of Obstetricians and Gynecologists	www.acog.org
Association of Women's Health, Obstetric and Neonatal Nurses	www.awhonn.org
The Center for Disease Control and Prevention	www.cdc.gov
March of Dimes	www.modimes.com
U.S. Food and Drug Administration	www.cfsan.fda.gov

index

Note: The italicized *f* or *t* following page numbers refer to figures and tables, respectively.

A

abdominal itching 41
abdominal muscles
  belly breathing and 47
  chair exercises 139-141
  crunches 119
  muscle pulls 118
  returning to normal 41
ACOG (American College
       of Obstetricians and
       Gynecologists) 71
active labor 167-168
acupressure points 24, 25, 27
aerobic activities 76. *See also*
       exercising to manage stress
afterbirth 170
alcohol consumption 2
alternating bridge 191
American College of Obstetricians and
       Gynecologists (ACOG) 71
anemia 113
ankle swelling 27, 32, 139
anxiety during pregnancy 31
appetite increase during pregnancy
       33
arm strengtheners 144-145

B

babies. *See* newborns
Babinski's sign 177
back, staying off of during second
       trimester 124-125
back discomfort
  exercising with a chair 133, 139-
       141
  postpartum phase 174-175
  during pregnancy 28
back muscles and belly breathing
       47-48
back protection 35-36
back strengtheners 133, 139-141
back stretch, wall-supported 16
balancing sunbird 8, 98
belly breathing 6
  chest wall activity reduction 48
  diaphragmatic breathing 46-47
  diaphragm strengthening 49-50
  finding your natural rhythm 50
  fitness ball exercises 115-116
  learning to use 47
  muscle strengthening 91
  rib cage and back muscles and
       47-48
belly dance 161
birth plan 149-151
blood pooling 19
blood pressure, low 26
blood sugar, low. *See* hypoglycemia
bound angle 18, 87
bowling 78
Braxton Hicks contractions 128
breast care and examination 38-40
breastfeeding and exercise 175
breastfeeding and weight loss 172
breath counting meditation 105-106
breathing
  belly. *See* belly breathing
  chair exercises 133
  exercises 51-52
  during labor 157
  postpartum exercise 188
  rates during pregnancy 30-31
bridges 190-191, 200
buttock strengtheners 141-143

C

caffeine 114
calcium
    deficiency causing leg cramps 26,
        127
    as a nausea relief 25
calcium-phosphorus imbalance 127
calf stretch 89, 137-139
cancer, breast 39
cancer, skin 40
carbohydrate consumption 56
cardiovascular fitness 67-68
carpal tunnel syndrome 28-29, 32,
    125
cat bows 91
catecholamines 156
cat stretch 139-140
chair exercises
    abdominal strengtheners 139-141
    arm strengtheners 144-145
    back strengtheners 133, 139-141
    breathing 133
    buttock strengtheners 141-143
    hip strengtheners 141-143
    hip stretch, sitting 136
    leg and calf stretches 137-139
    neck stretches 134
    posture 133
    shoulder stretch 135
    torso stretch, sitting 135
chair pose 95
chakras 107, 108f
child's pose 48f
cholasma 40
Christiansen, Ingrid 66
circulation, sluggish 26-28
colic 178-179
constipation 25
contractions
    active labor 167-168
    early labor 165-167
    pushing during labor 168-170
cool-down 19-20, 197
core conditioning
    balancing sunbird 8
    belly breathing 6
    flamingo 7
    half crescent moon 9

importance of 5-6
    Kegel exercises 11
    rounded cat stretch 6-7
    spinal twists 10-11
crying, excessive 178-179
cycling 80
cycling, stationary 76

D

darkening of the skin 40
delivery. *See* labor and delivery
dental care 38
depression, postpartum 173
depression during pregnancy 31
diabetes, gestational 69
diaphragmatic breathing 46-47, 50
diaphragm strengthening 49-50
digestive problems during pregnancy
    24-25, 114
discomfort during labor
    active labor 167-168
    breathing 157
    early labor 165-167
    exercises to cope with labor. *See*
        exercising during labor
    massage use 163-164
    music and relaxation 164
    pain management 154-156
    positioning 158-160
    relaxation 156-157, 165
    visualization 157
    water 158
discomforts during pregnancy 23t
    appetite increase 33
    back protection 35-36
    breast care and examination 38-
        40
    breathing rates 30-31
    digestive problems 24-25, 114
    emotional challenges 31
    foot care 37-38
    joint protection 32
    muscular aches and pains 28-29
    pelvic concerns 30
    rest requirements 42-43
    skin care and examination 40-41
    sluggish circulation 26-28
    teeth care 38

temperature sensitivity 32
water retention 32
double-foot touch 190

E
early labor 165-167
eating plan 55-56. *See also* nutrition
    during pregnancy
emotional challenges during
    pregnancy 31
endorphins 156
episiotomy 147-148
exercise instructors 80-81
exercise intensity 79
exercising after delivery 175-176
exercising during labor
    belly dance 161
    lion pose 162
    shoulder stretch 160-161*f*
    squatting 163
    wall-assisted body stretch 162
exercising during pregnancy
    for athletes 79-81
    benefits from 66
    eating schedule and 57, 146
    effects on length and type of
        delivery 66
    first trimester. *See* fitness ball
        exercises
    maternal response to. *See*
        maternal response to
        exercise
    muscle strengthening. *See* muscle
        strengthening exercises
    overtraining symptoms 73
    physiological considerations 71-72
    safety and 74-75
    stretching. *See* stretching before
        exercise, pregnancy
    third trimester. *See* chair exercises
    types of exercise 75-79
    workout schedule 100-101
exercising postpartum
    alternating bridge 191
    with the baby. *See* exercising with
        baby
    basic bridge 190
    basics 186-187

breathing 188
cool-down 197
double-foot touch 190
heel slides 189
hundreds 192
oblique strengtheners 195
pelvic tilt, lying 188
progressive bridge 191
rolling 194
roll-ups 193
side kicks 196
single-foot touch 189
single-leg kick 195
single-leg stretch 194
swimmer 196
exercising to manage stress
    cool-down 19-20
    core conditioning. *See* core
        conditioning
    flexibility improvement. *See*
        stretching before exercise,
        pre-pregnancy
    non-walking aerobic activities 5
    walking 4-5
exercising with baby
    back strengthener 199
    bridges 200
    downward facing baby 200
    kiss the baby 199
    presses 198
    sit-ups 198
    tips 197
eyedropper breathing exercise 52

F
family fitness 201
fatigue 114
fetal movements, counting 127-128
first trimester
    exercising. *See* fitness ball
        exercises
    morning sickness 112
    tips for coping 112-114
fish consumption during pregnancy
    62-63
fitness ball exercises
    abdominal crunches 119
    balancing 120

fitness ball exercises   *(continued)*
  belly breathing 115-116
  benefits from 114-115
  hip circles 116
  oblique crunches 119
  side stretches 120-121
  single-leg balance 117
  single-leg balance with torso
      rotation 117
  torso turns 116
  walk-outs 118
flamingo 7
flexibility improvement. *See*
    stretching before exercise,
    pre-pregnancy
folic acid 61
food dairy 57, 58*f*
food pyramid 3*f*, 56*f*
foot care 37-38
forward bend, standing 17

G

gallant response 177
garland pose 16, 86
gas in a baby 179
gazing meditation 106
genetic counseling 2
gestational diabetes 69
golfing 78

H

half crescent moon 9
HCG (human chorionic gonadotropin)
    112
headaches 27
heartburn 25, 146
heart palpitations 26
heat stress 69
heel slides 189
hemorrhoids 25
hip circles 116
hip flexor/monkey stretch 14
hip strengtheners 141-143
hip stretch, sitting 90, 136
horseback riding 74, 79
hospital, when to go 166
human chorionic gonadotropin (HCG)
    112
humming meditation 107

hundreds exercise 192
hypoglycemia 55-56, 57

I

incline plane exercise 92
inferior vena cava 124
infertility 4
in-line skating 78
inner thigh lift, sidelying 97
insulin sensitivity 69
iron supplements 61

J

jogging 76
joint protection 32

K

Kegel exercises 11, 116, 175

L

labor and delivery
  active labor 167-168
  afterbirth 170
  early labor 165-167
  exercise and. *See* exercising during
      labor
  pushing 168-170
  relieving discomfort during. *See*
      discomfort during labor
labor bag 150
lateral stretch, sitting 87
leg cramps 26-27, 126
leg exercises
  inner thigh lift, sidelying 97
  leg extension 12, 84, 88
  leg stretch, elevated 13, 17
  quadriceps stretch 13
  single-foot touch 189
  single-leg balance 117
  single-leg kick 195
  single-leg stretch 194
leg stretch, chair exercises 137-139
lifting procedure 36
light-headedness 125
lion pose 162
lunges 36, 37*f*, 94

M

making love after delivery 184-186

making love during pregnancy 129-130

mammography 3

mantra meditation 106

mask of pregnancy 40

massage for infants 180-182

massage use during labor 163-164

maternal response to exercise
cardiovascular 67-68
heat stress handling 69
insulin sensitivity 69
labor and delivery and 71
maternal discomforts and 70
metabolic capacity 69
musculoskeletal function 69-70
positive attitude 71, 72
stamina and energy and 68

medication during delivery 151

meditation
benefits from 104
breath counting 105-106
gazing 106
getting started 104-105
humming 107
mantra 106
om 106
preparing for labor 108-110
rainbow 107, 108*f*

melanoma 40

metabolic capacity 69

methylmercury 62

modified mermaid 93

monkey stretch 14, 83

morning sickness 112. *See also* nausea

Moro reflex 176-177

muscle strengthening exercises
balancing sunbird 98
belly breathing 91
cat bows 91
chair pose 95
incline plane 92
inner thigh lift, sidelying 97
lunges 94
modified mermaid 93
sit-backs 99
stork pose 94
sunbird pose 98

wall push-ups 92

warrior poses 96, 97*f*

muscular aches and pains 28-29

music and relaxation 164

N

nausea 24-25, 112, 114

neck relaxer 88

neck stretches 134

nerve compression syndrome 28-29, 32, 125

newborns
baby's temperament 184
exercising with. *See* exercising with baby
infant massage 180-182
reflexes 176-177
schedules 177-178
states of consciousness 178*t*

nostril breathing, alternate 51-52

nutritional habits, pre-pregnancy 2, 3*f*

nutrition during postpartum phase 172, 173*t*

nutrition during pregnancy
eating before exercise 57
eating plan 55-56, 57*t*
food dairy 57, 58*f*
foods to avoid 62-63
key nutrients 59*t*
for vegetarians 61, 62*f*
vitamins and minerals 58, 59*t*
weight gain 54-55, 60

O

oblique crunches 119

oblique strengtheners 195

om meditation 106

overtraining symptoms 73

P

pain management during labor 154-156

palmer grasp 176

palpitations, heart 26

partner's health 3

pelvic concerns during pregnancy 30

pelvic tilt, lying 188

perineal massage 148-149
phosphorus 26, 127
Pilates 76-77
plantar grasp 176
positioning during labor 158-160
post-delivery adjustments. *See also* postpartum phase
  baby's temperament and 184
  exercising. *See* exercising postpartum
  lifetime family fitness 201
  sexual health and 184-186
postpartum depression 173
postpartum phase. *See also* post-delivery adjustments
  back discomfort 174-175
  depression and 173
  exercising after delivery 175-176
  infant massage 180-182
  newborn excessive crying 178-179
  newborn reflexes 176-177
  newborn schedules 177-178
  newborn states of consciousness 178t
  nutrition during 172, 173t
posture 33-34, 50, 133
prana 51
preeclampsia 70
premature labor 128-129
prenatal vitamins 24, 58
pre-pregnancy health
  assessment 2-4
  exercise and stress management. *See* exercising to manage stress
pressure points
  to relieve headaches 27
  to relieve nausea 25
progesterone
  breathing rates and 30
  digestive problems and 25
  low blood pressure and 26
progressive bridge 191
pruritic urticarial papules (PUPP) 41
pubic area pressure 136
pushing during labor 168-170

Q
quadriceps stretch 13, 85
quickening 127

R
racquetball 78
rainbow meditation 107, 108f
relaxation techniques during labor 156-157, 165
relaxin 32, 69-70
relief strategies for common discomforts. *See* discomforts during pregnancy
rest requirements 42-43
rib cage and belly breathing 47-48
rolling exercise 194
roll-ups exercise 193
rounded cat stretch 6-7
running 76, 80

S
safety and exercising during pregnancy 74-75
sciatica in pregnancy 146-147
scuba diving 74, 78
sea bands 24
seafood consumption during pregnancy 62
secondhand smoke 3
second trimester
  fetal movements counting 127-128
  making love during pregnancy 129-130
  premature labor 128-129
  reclaiming your energy 126-127
  staying off your back 124-125
serving sizes for foods 57t
sexual health after delivery 184-186
shoulder stretch 15, 83
  chair exercises 135
  exercising during labor 160-161f
  to relieve discomfort 29
side kicks 196
side stretches 120-121
Simethicone drops 179
sit-backs 99

skin care and examination 40-41
sky diving 74
sleeplessness during pregnancy 31
smoking, pre-pregnancy 2
snorkeling 78
snow skiing 78
spinal twists 10-11
spine rotation 89
spinning classes 72
squatting 14, 86, 163
stability 5
stamina and energy 68
startle reflex in newborns 177
states of consciousness, newborn 178t
step aerobics 76
stepping reflex in newborns 177
stork pose 94
stress, pre-pregnancy. *See* exercising to manage stress
stretching before exercise, pregnancy
    bound angle 87
    calf 89
    frequency 81
    garland pose 86
    hip, sitting 90
    lateral, sitting 87
    leg extension 84
    leg extension, sidelying 88
    monkey stretch 83
    neck relaxer 88
    quadriceps stretch 85
    shoulder stretch 83
    spine rotation 89
    squatting 86
    torso stretch, standing 82
    triangle pose, modified 90
stretching before exercise, pre-pregnancy
    back stretch, wall-supported 16
    bound angle 18
    forward bend, standing 17
    garland pose 16
    hip flexor/monkey stretch 14
    importance of 12
    leg extension 12
    leg stretch, elevated 17

quadriceps stretch 13
shoulder stretch 15
squatting 14
swan 18
torso stretch, standing 15
stretch marks 41
stroller posture 174
sunbird pose 98
supplements, nutritional 58, 61
surfing 78
swan stretch 18
swimmer exercise 196
swimming 66, 76, 80
swollen ankles 27, 32, 139

T
teeth care 38
temperature sensitivity 32
tennis 78
tetanus-diphtheria (Td) booster 3
third trimester
    birth plan 149-151
    episiotomy pros and cons 147-148
    exercising during. *See* chair exercises
    perineal massage 148-149
    sciatica in pregnancy 146-147
    thinking positively 132
    when to go to the hospital 166
three-part breathing 52
torso stretch, sitting 135
torso stretch, standing 15, 82
torso turns 116, 117
transition phase of labor 167-168
triangle pose, modified 90

U
urinary tract infections 30

V
vaccines 3
varicose veins 26
vegetarian nutrition during pregnancy 61, 62f
visualization during labor 157
Vitamin C 26
vitamins and minerals, prenatal 24, 58, 59t

vomiting 24

W

walking 4-5, 75-76
walking reflex in newborns 177
walk-outs 118
wall-assisted exercises
   back stretch 16
   during labor 162
   push-ups 92
warrior poses 96, 97f
water pitcher breathing exercise 52
water retention 32
water skiing 78
water use during labor 158

weight gain
   during pregnancy 54-55
   tips for avoiding 60
weight lifting 80
weight loss, postpartum 172, 187
weight training 77-78
workout schedule 100-101
wrist sensitivity 7, 125

X

Xrays, pre-pregnancy 3

Y

yoga 77

about the author

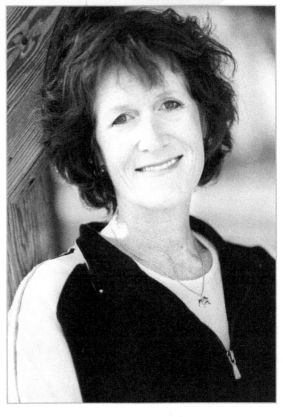

Bonnie Berk, RN, is the founder of Motherwell and a childbirth education specialist with more than 25 years of experience working in the obstetrical and women's health fields. She is a pioneer in the field of pre- and postnatal fitness, as proven with the success of the Motherwell program. This program is offered through more than 100 hospitals and fitness centers in the United States and abroad.

Berk is an author, speaker, and consultant to a broad range of institutions addressing the special needs of women before, during, and after pregnancy. She is a frequent TV and radio talk show guest, has been featured on the Discovery Channel, and serves as the fitness expert on the Harrisburg ABC affiliate, WHTM-TV 27, on the Daybreak Show. She has given presentations throughout the United States and has written numerous articles that have been featured in *Baby Talk*, *Pregnancy*, *Vogue*, *Shape*, *Fitness*, and many other consumer and trade publications. Berk has also produced two award-winning videos, *Motherwell Exercise Video for Pregnant Women* and *Motherwell Yoga Video for Expectant Moms*. In addition, she is a certified master personal fitness trainer through the IDEA Health and Fitness Association, a registered yoga teacher through Yoga Alliance, and a Pilates instructor certified by American Muscle and Fitness, Institute of Fitness Training.

Berk lives in Carlisle, Pennsylvania, and enjoys scuba diving, inline skating, and hiking. She can be reached through her Web site, www.motherwellfitness.com.

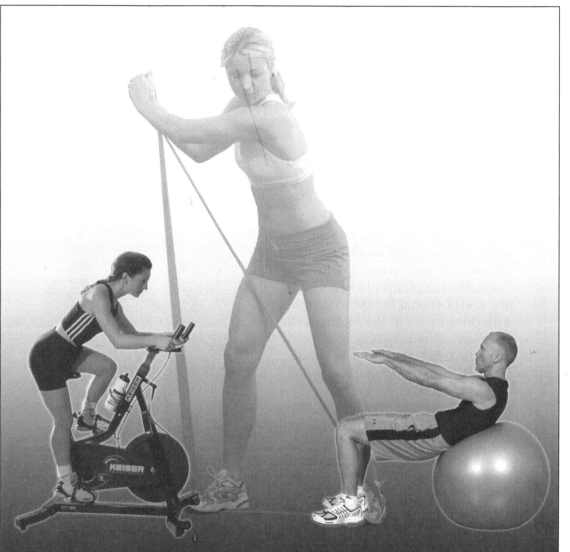

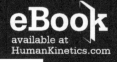